# CHRIS
# BASTEN PhD

help
solutions
anger
anxiety
alliance flexibility
response
thoughts individual management

# THE ART

worry
sadness
mindful

psychotherapy

behaviour mood phobia schemas feelings

# OF CBT

habits mind think
anxious

fear motivation engagement

cognitive emotions

## Individualised strategies to respond to common obstacles in therapy

brain aware actions

treatment

**AUSTRALIAN**ACADEMIC**PRESS**

First published 2019 by:
Australian Academic Press Group Pty. Ltd.
www.australianacademicpress.com.au

A catalogue record for this
book is available from the
National Library of Australia

ISBN    9781925644302 (paperback)
ISBN    9781925644319 (ebook)

**Disclaimer**
Every effort has been made in preparing this work to provide information based on accepted standards and practice at the time of publication. The publisher and author, however, make no warranties of any kind of psychological outcome relating to use of this work and disclaim all responsibility or liability for direct or consequential damages resulting from any use of the material contained in this work.

Publisher: Stephen May

Copy editing: Rhonda McPherson

Cover design: Jemima Ung

Typesetting: Australian Academic Press

Printing: Lightning Source

# Acknowledgments

This book is a coalescence of many years of clinical training and practice. I am very grateful to the supervisors and colleagues who have helped me develop some skills and knowledge and to my clients for providing lessons in the finer points of therapy. I am indebted to the editorial assistance of Melissa Franks and Kirsten Abbott as well as the team at Australian Academic Press for rendering the ideas more readable.

# Contents

Acknowledgments ........................................................................................ iii

About the Author ...................................................................................... ix

Preface .................................................................................................... xi

**Chapter 1: Three case studies** ................................................................. 1

    Amanda: A 31-year-old single woman experiencing panic attacks ....................... 1

    Neil: 53-year-old married man with depression ..................................... 3

    Monica: 21-year-old woman with social anxiety, anxiety attacks and worry that
    causes a sleep disturbance ......................................................................... 4

**Chapter 2: Tailoring your formulations** ................................................. 7

    Theoretical context ............................................................................... 7

    Tips on developing helpful formulations ................................................ 11

    Highlights and take-home messages ..................................................... 31

**Chapter 3: Developing, managing and using the therapeutic relationship** ...... 33

    What is the therapeutic relationship and alliance? .............................. 33

    How important is the TA and relationship? ......................................... 35

    Therapist qualities and skills that deepen the bond and therapeutic alliance .... 36

    Ways to monitor and measure the strength of your TA ...................... 43

    Noticing and managing ruptures ........................................................ 44

    Case studies ........................................................................................ 48

    Working on your therapeutic relationships ........................................ 50

    Is there a risk of overemphasising the TA? ......................................... 52

    Highlights and take-home messages ..................................................... 53

**Chapter 4: Understanding and maintaining motivational dynamics** ....... 55

    What is motivation? ............................................................................. 57

    Understanding readiness to change .................................................... 60

    Common reasons for ambivalence ...................................................... 64

    Key strategies to build motivation ...................................................... 66

    Important caveats ............................................................................... 82

    Highlights and take-home messages ..................................................... 83

**Chapter 5: Working with all levels of cognition** ..............................**85**

How to help clients identify their emotions
and thoughts for cognitive therapy ......................................87

Accessing automatic thoughts...........................................88

Hot cognitions ...............................................................91

Implicit assumptions .......................................................91

Metacognitions...............................................................93

Core beliefs....................................................................93

Summary: Identifying the right cognition to challenge ...........97

Highlights and take-home messages ..................................99

**Chapter 6: Creative behavioural experiments**.............................**101**

The nine elements of a good behavioural experiment ...........102

Troubleshooting with behavioural experiments....................110

Highlights and take-home messages ..................................113

**Chapter 7: Getting on track and staying
on track: Avoiding therapeutic drift** ...........................**115**

Responsibility................................................................116

Staying on track with homework ......................................117

How does therapeutic drift occur?....................................119

Highlights and take-home messages ..................................127

**References** ....................................................................**129**

**Appendix A: Four Visual Analogue Scales for Assessing Willingness** ...........**137**

**Appendix B: Layers of Cognition — Blank Client Worksheet**......................**139**

**Appendix C: Worksheet to Practice Identifying Cognitions**........................**141**

**Appendix D:**

Part A. Client Handout on How to Learn Cognitive Therapy.............................143

Part B. A Brief Formula for Thought Challenging.................................146

Part C. Practicing Cognitive Therapy at an Effective Level .................148

**Appendix E: Example of a Behavioural Experiment Worksheet** ....................151

**Appendix F: Client Worksheet for the End of Each Consultation** ..................153

**Appendix G: Handout for Clients on Effective Therapy** ..................................155

Dr Chris Basten is a highly experienced clinical psychologist with particular interests in health psychology, eating disorders and motivational interviewing. He has completed degrees in psychology at the University of NSW (Bachelor of Arts) and the University of Sydney (Master of Psychology and PhD). Chris has more than 25 years' experience in clinical settings including private practice, vocational rehabilitation and public hospitals. For the last 10 years he has focused on his own practice and training psychologists and other health professionals CBT and motivational interviewing.

The greater the artist, the greater the doubt. Perfect confidence
is granted to the less talented as a consolation prize.

Robert Hughes

This book is aimed at clinicians who are comfortably familiar with the theory and practice of cognitive–behaviour therapy (CBT) and who wish to tailor their treatment to individual clients more powerfully, while still adhering to core CBT as an evidenced-based treatment (EBT). References are made to certain theoretical models and treatment principles without explaining these core constructs in any detail. It is assumed that the reader has had some training in the theory and clinical application of:

- Key elements of a cognitive-behavioural assessment

- The use of self-monitoring as an assessment process and as a therapeutic tool

- The use of psychoeducation as therapeutic tool

- The use of clinical formulations in the way the clinician understands a set of presenting problems and shares a rationale for treatment with the client

- Cognitive restructuring for common conditions such as panic disorder, generalised anxiety disorder, social anxiety, phobias, self-esteem issues, eating disorders and depression

- Common behavioural interventions, such as behavioural activation for depression, prolonged exposure for trauma, systematic desensitisation for anxiety conditions and behavioural experiments.

The aim is to enable the clinician to adapt their application of cognitive therapy principles in response to the common challenges of everyday practice. The common challenges that the cognitive–behavioural (CB) therapist encounters include:

- emotional avoidance

- resistance within therapy

- ambivalence towards change

- failure to do homework

- missed appointments, and

- keeping a client focused on goals and a therapy agenda.

Accordingly, following the introduction of three core case studies in Chapter 1, each of the remaining six chapters presents the reader with some methodological solutions for challenges and forms of resistance. These six domains of clinical practice are known to many CB therapists, and yet they are seldom written about collectively in one resource.

The figure on the facing page illustrates the chief components that make CBT creative, individually tailored and responsive to common clinical challenges. At the centre of this model lies the clinical case formulation that includes the presenting problem, the contributing and maintaining factors and any other element that informs the therapy and adds understanding for your client. It is argued throughout this book that the formulations that you use with your client needs to evolve with therapy progression and can incorporate all the factors that comprise the rest of the book. Therefore, the formulations that you use in therapy are revisited in each chapter hereafter.

Looking beyond the centrality of the case formulation, the therapeutic relationship in the left-top corner is viewed as the obvious place to start and so is the first of the domains to be addressed. The vast majority of clients, at some points in the therapy process, will need some conscious effort to increase their motivation and willingness to do the tasks that will

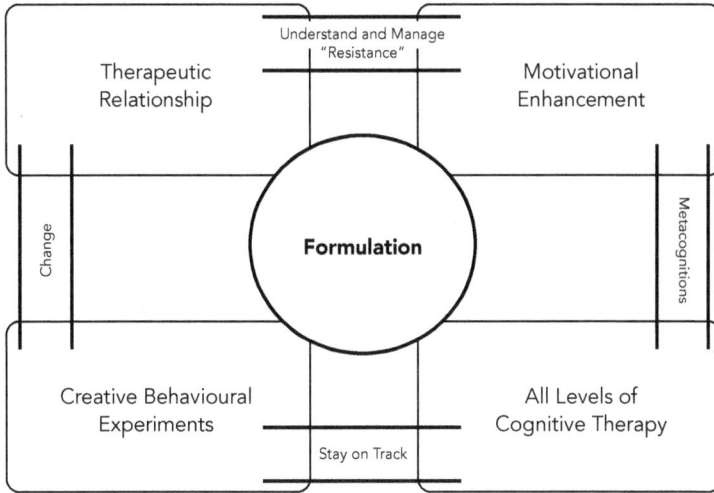

A formulation-centric problem-solving plan for CBT.

lead to change. The way this is linked to the formulation as well as the therapeutic relationship and good cognitive therapy is illustrated in the Figure above and explained through the relevant chapters. It helps both the therapeutic relationship and the motivational dynamics if the clinician understands and can manage different types of resistance.

Cognitive therapy needs to cover all the types and depths of cognition, from metacognitions, though automatic thoughts, the hidden assumptions, personal rules and stable beliefs down to one's early maladaptive schemas. The metacognitions are drawn as a bridge between motivation and cognition mainly because a lot of metacognitions will erode willingness to work hard in treatment, as explained in Chapter 5. Behavioural change strategies and deliberate experimentation constitute some of the most powerful methods to change what our clients think about themselves and the world, which thus enables emotional change.

Finally, in order to do all this well, the client needs to stay on track, and it is the clinician's responsibility to identify when either they or the client is drifting away from the therapy tasks that will actually get the client better.

The book takes a formulation-centric view on clinical problem solving. Some common challenges are discussed and each chapter adds extra detail and ideas to overcome specific problems. For instance, Chapter 4 outlines how the case formulation can enrich the therapeutic relationship and reduce the likelihood of breaches in the alliance. Chapter 5 illustrates how to add motivational dynamics to a case formulation and Chapter 6 incorporates levels of cognition that the client will need to keep in mind but will not immediately be aware of.

The 'art' of CBT does not imply that it is more art than skill; the art lies in studying its components and methodically, deliberately getting them as right as we can. As Vincent van Gogh is credited to have said: 'Great things are not done by impulse, but by a series of small things brought together'.

# Chapter 1

# Three case studies

Each of the major themes in this book will be illustrated with cases, and three people presenting for psychological therapy are described here for that purpose. These three 'cases' are not real clients or people but are fictional and have been constructed for teaching purposes from a combination of people who typically seek help.

### Amanda: A 31-year-old single woman experiencing panic attacks

Amanda presents with fairly typical panic disorder. She has frequent acute anxiety attacks, especially when outside the comfort zones of her home, her two close friends' apartments and the roads on the way to those apartments. She feels unable to take a train or a bus or drive to a suburb that she is not familiar with. Her panic attacks are characterised by an overwhelming feeling that she is going to collapse or faint. Her legs 'feel like jelly' and she feels that she cannot catch her breath properly. At times, she feels that her heart might stop beating. Therefore, if standing, she feels that she must sit down and, if sitting, she worries that if she might collapse if she stands. During these attacks, Amanda also feels 'out of control'. Questioned about this, Amanda explains, 'Well, I try to calm my mind and I can't. I try to calm my body and I can't. I can't breathe even though I try with all my might. I can't even focus my attention where I want it. I can't control my body or my mind, so I'm not in control.' She has recently started to worry that, while anxious and therefore not in control she could assault someone or cause a fatal accident. She worries about this between panic attacks.

Her goal in therapy is to stop her panic attacks. Amanda said she would do anything to stop these episodes from happening again.

The therapist has designed a treatment for Amanda that includes: psychoeducation about the fight–flight response, panic attacks and how they are safe, as well as the role of hyperventilation in a panic attack and therefore the potential help of slow breathing. The main focus, though, is on her fear that something terrible will happen if she panics (fainting, heart failure or losing control and causing injury to someone). For this, the therapist asks Amanda to list and reflect on all the existing personal evidence she has that anxiety is safe and then they collaboratively, systematically gather new evidence that her fears will not come true through exposure-based behavioural experiments. The therapist explains that these crucial experiments will help change her fear of anxiety by altering her beliefs about the dangerousness of anxiety and perhaps also through getting used to the sensations of anxiety. Finally, the therapist suggests that she starts travelling to places that she needs to go for better functioning, such as catching a train, driving a few blocks further than she feels comfortable, and so on. With help, Amanda is able to establish a 'fear hierarchy' and the therapist explains how she can tackle one or two very small goals each week to progress towards her bigger therapy goals.

Amanda seems to comprehend the psychoeducation — she can repeat it back to you and she agrees that out of her hundreds of anxiety attacks, even the severe ones, that she has never collapsed, died or attacked anyone. She is willing to do some interoceptive exposure with you in session but her fear levels remain very high and her *danger expectancies* do not alter over time. She is very reluctant to repeat the interceptive exposure on her own at home and she very rarely follows the homework tasks of driving a little more each week according to the fear-hierarchy that you established for her agoraphobic avoidance.

Amanda starts reflecting on how long the treatment is taking. She blames herself for being 'stupid' and 'not trying hard enough'. She asks at least once every session if you are annoyed with her. She says things like, 'I know you must be SO frustrated with me. Will you keep treating me?'. Despite reassurance that this is not the case, she keeps asking the same thing over subsequent consultations. She also states that she is worried this constant need for reassurance is annoying.

## Neil: 53-year-old married man with depression

Neil requests help for depressed mood. His symptoms include sleep disturbance with early morning waking, increased irritability and feeling despondent and sad much of every day. He reports that it has been a few years since he felt any pleasure, interest or enthusiasm. He thinks about dying but worries about how his two daughters would cope if he completed suicide and has vowed to himself that he will not act on these thoughts. He denies psychomotor retardation. He denies excessive drinking or other substance use.

During the assessment phase, Neil suggests several reasons why he feels consistently unhappy. He said that his wife's career means that she is often tired and they do not have time to spend together. He was happier when she took time away from work and when his two daughters were much younger. His work as a chief operations officer features high volume and deadlines. There is conflict at work because of the high demands that he places on his team and the managers that report to him. He has two daughters, one with severe depression and dramatic mood swings and one who is married and functioning well. The one with the mood disturbance often calls him for support and often says that she feels suicidal. She does not work and Neil is paying all her rent, all her food and telephone bills and a few hundred dollars a week to allow her to go to the hair and eyebrow salon as often as she needs to prevent her depression from worsening. The other daughter resents her sister (for what she sees as emotional manipulation of her father) and her father (whom she sees as being too weak to decline her constant demands for money). He has been lying to his wife and other daughter about how much money she receives and he is worried that it will deplete his retirement savings.

At session four, his wife is sitting with him in the waiting room and says that she would like to come in. You check with Neil, who indicates that he wants his wife to join the appointment. She asks if Neil has been entirely honest about his drinking, which is every day of the week and always at least a bottle of wine to himself. On weekends she has found that he is drinking scotch surreptitiously before dinner. She has tried to discuss his drinking, as it makes her very worried about his wellbeing and the way it affects their relationship.

During session six, Neil reveals to you that his 36-year-old personal assistant at work left last year. He had a sexual and emotionally intense relationship with her for several years. He said that he let her believe that he would leave his wife, which he did think about. She increased her requests to know when this would happen, saying that she wanted to start a family of their own, at which time Neil told her that that was never going to happen and he wanted to stay with his family. He feels guilty for preventing her from having a chance at a different relationship or starting her own family, and this guilt, as well as the rupture of not seeing her, contributed to his depression worsening quite severely six months ago.

## Monica: 21-year-old woman with social anxiety, anxiety attacks and worry that causes a sleep disturbance

Monica advises she lives at home with her parents, is studying at college and has recently reduced her study load by 50% because her anxiety prevents her from coping. Her parents feel this is due more to 'laziness' than anxiety. They say she does not seem anxious around them or other family. However, Monica explains that she avoids places where she predicts she might become the centre of attention and thereby become anxious.

There has been a fluctuation in the severity of her anxiety disorder. At the beginning of her final year at school, aged 17 years, Monica started to have anxiety attacks and frequently asked to stay at home from school. The anxiety began with any presentation she had to give but soon was happening on a daily basis. Initially, her mother agreed but then organised the school counsellor and a private psychologist to provide intensive treatment. She also started to drive Monica to school each day and reduced her responsibilities at home (such as doing her own ironing and feeding the family dogs). A few months after that year at school, Monica's anxiety seemed to halve in intensity but it was triggered again when she started college. Now is her final year at college, and her anxiety attacks and worry have intensified enough to require treatment.

The therapist teaches her core cognitive therapy: learning to notice her mood states as the observer, then seeking out the thoughts and assumptions that drive the worry or acute anxiety. Monica is then taught how to dispute the automatic thoughts and the hidden assumptions. With time, she is encouraged to use more 'cognitive defusion' than 'disputation' because the same thoughts keep recurring in similar stressful situations. Rather than teaching her how to relax in social situations (e.g., slow breathing or distraction or reassuring self-talk), Monica is encouraged to view her fearful predictions as unhelpful and inaccurate cognitions that are not facts and not ever likely to happen. Consultation time is devoted to helping her to reflect on the existing evidence that her worst fears have never yet come true. She is asked to reflect on how her avoidance to date prevents her from testing and disproving some of her fears and discovering that alternatives may be true. Homework involves her learning to monitor her thoughts and remain the detached, sceptical observer. When it is time to do a behavioural experiment together in a treatment consultation, Monica says that she is not ready and wants to discuss other things, like her friend posting an ugly photo of her on social media.

The therapist wonders what factors might contribute to Monica avoiding active treatment and notes that anxiety was at its worst in the final year of high school and the final year of tertiary education — times of maturity transition. In response to further specific questions about maturity, Monica admits that she is scared of the thought of being an adult. She is reassessed for trauma, especially unwanted sexual advances or abuse, even though during the initial phase of assessment she denied any such problems. Again, she is sure that this is not the case and then says that she feels like such a fraud for being 'so screwed up even though nothing awful ever happened to me'. In fact, she says she was provided a sheltered life, which causes the therapist to consider formation pathways for schemas, and so screens for certain core beliefs. Whereupon, Monica reveals that she feels completely incompetent socially and in terms of daily living skills. She has never told anyone, including her last psychologist, but she worries most days about (a) people discovering how useless she is in her character and (b) coping with life's challenges that seem to increase in complexity with every year that she is alive.

# Chapter 2

# Tailoring your formulations

Perhaps the most compelling reason for utilizing a case
formulation is to anticipate roadblocks and noncompliance.

(Leahy, 2003, p. 345)

The broad focus of the book is on solving common problems that arise in therapy and this is true also for this section. This chapter starts by outlining the essence of a useful formulation but the emphasis is on how to ensure that each formulation is tailored and purposeful. Some common challenges are discussed and each subsequent chapter adds extra detail and ideas to overcome specific problems.

## Theoretical context

There is some debate in the literature about whether a clinician should structure therapy according to a diagnosis or an individual case formulation (ICF; Dudley, Kuyken, & Padesky, 2011; Hallam, 2013). One argument against an ICF approach is that manualised treatments for a diagnosis (such as social phobia or panic disorder) are of known effectiveness and when the clinician decides to alter that treatment at all, such as to tailor it to an individual, then they are no longer providing evidence-based treatment (EBT). There is also some empirical evidence that personal clinical judgement, even by experienced clinicians, is not superior to protocol-based formulations and treatments (Grove, Zald, Lebow, Snitz, & Nelson, 2000). What is more, there is little evidence yet that formulations are reliable and can be reproduced (e.g., by a majority of therapists for the one client). Others argue that using a *case formulation* instead of a *diagnosis* can lead to clinical errors, such as the missing of a diagnosis, and therefore poor outcomes for our clients.

In response to the EBT argument, the clinician can bring a nuanced formulation to the treatment process and still adhere to known treatments. This is explained and illustrated throughout the chapter. With regard to the importance of making a diagnosis, the approach advocated here is that a clinician will indeed do a thorough assessment that will permit them to explore all possible diagnoses and differential diagnoses. Once one or more diagnoses have been made, then the first formulation can start to be established. This permits a functional analysis of the client's behaviour that focuses on the intrapersonal, family and social contributing factors and highlights the maintaining factors keeping this person stuck in their distress.

An evolution of this functional approach is proposed by Hayes et al. (1996) in which they advocate that common processes of aetiology and maintenance ('functional diagnostic dimensions') should be the basis for research and clinical practice. This is one of the underpinnings of a transdiagnostic approach. Several authors have identified factors that serve as common causes and maintaining factors for several conditions (that is, they are transdiagnostic). For instance, Ingram (1990) and Woodruff-Borden, Brothers and Lister (2001) have suggested that self-focused attention is common across many disorders. Hayes Wilson, Gifford, Follette & Strosahl (1996) have shown that experiential avoidance of feelings, memories and thoughts is a powerful maintaining factor of distress generally and is a process that is common to many diagnosable disorders. Egan, Wade & Shafran (2011) have presented evidence that unhealthy perfectionism is a cognitive process that disposes a person to several different conditions such as depression, eating disorders and some anxiety states. Fairburn, Cooper and Shafran (2003) have provided an empirically supported model that all eating disorders are caused and maintained by common factors (such as excessive focus on controlling weight and shape in self-evaluation and the consequences of dieting) and so a treatment that targets the common beliefs, behaviours and cognitive errors can be effectively applied to bulimia, anorexia and their variants. McEvoy and Mahoney (2013) have noted how intolerance of uncertainty and negative metacognitive beliefs serve as transdiagnostic mediators of several anxiety disorders. Harvey, Watkins, Mansell, & Shafran (2004) have conducted a comprehensive review of the literature on cognitive and behavioural processes that are common across disorders.

In response to such findings, Barlow and colleagues have collated several factors that appear to be common to much psychological distress and have developed a 'unified' CBT package that is readily mastered by clinicians and can be used in health services to treat the underlying mechanisms of psychological disorders, rather than treating each disorder in sequence (Barlow, Farchione, Bullis, & Gallagher, 2017; Farchione et al., 2012).

The fact that the majority of clients present with more than one condition and that there are common vulnerability factors across disorders lends support to a functional or case formulation approach. The position recommended in this book is that the clinician ought to follow EBT's as much as the presentation permits and adherence to a known manual tends to deliver better client outcomes than experienced clinician judgement (Grove et al., 2000). These procedural manuals, however, do not manage comorbidity well and typically have no guidance on how to deal with resistance and ambivalence in clients. A rare but excellent exception is the Maudsley Anorexia Nervosa Treatment for Adults protocol in which intense ambivalence about recovery is a key feature of the underpinning theoretical model (Treasure & Schmidt, 2013) and the treatment manual includes specific motivational enhancement techniques for the client as well as the therapist (Schmidt, Startup, & Treasure, 2018).

Furthermore, when a good case formulation is employed, the client will feel as if the treatment is tailored to them, aiding the therapeutic alliance and therefore the degree to which the client will work hard. One can employ an ICF and still adhere very closely to a manualised version of therapy (Wilson, 1996). As Hallam states in his very helpful account of ICF's, 'However much a general model of therapeutic change has been supported by evidence, it is its detailed translation for the individual that is of paramount importance' (Hallam, 2013; p. 2). Sketching a formulation for your client in their words and using personal examples of maintaining factors (rather than a generic phrase such as 'avoidance') will help the client feel that you have been listening and that this treatment is in response to their needs and their issues. All the while, the clinician knows that they are borrowing from and adapting the generic model and have all the treatment implications in mind.

An important additional argument is that therapists are not always treating a specific diagnostic condition (like social phobia; obsessive-compulsive disorder [OCD]; panic disorder) but are often required to respond to requests for help with 'problems' or nondiagnostic distress for which there will not be a therapy manual nor a known theoretical model. The core question that we work through with our client is a variation on the cardinal question 'Why is this problem causing this level of distress and impairment in this client at this time?'. And, as noted already, most of these presenting problems coexist with other problems and perhaps with a diagnosable condition for which there is an EBT procedure. Thus, wherever it is possible, a clinician should endeavour to use a theory-driven and evidence-based approach for a discrete clinical problem. In the many instances where this is not readily possible, then the skilled therapist will use the knowledge and skills that they possess to do treatments that (a) are derived from a theoretical model, (b) incorporate elements of EBTs, and (c) are grounded on an individually tailored formulation of the problem(s) that the client wants to work on.

As an example, if a client presents with body dysmorphic disorder, generalised anxiety disorder and concurrent depression, a clinician may not adopt all of the manualised therapy for each or one of these conditions. Rather, they may attempt a formulation which encompasses several of these factors and negotiate collaboratively with the client which or their issues makes sense to tackle first. Having made enough progress on that issue, it may be desirable or even necessary to shift the focus temporarily to another issue, all the while using well-established therapies such as cognitive restructuring and exposure-based procedures, incorporating that individual's circumstances and capacities. The clinician is then using interventions known to work but could be said to have now departed from manualised treatment. This has been termed 'evidence-informed treatments', which are widely accepted as pragmatic and ethically accepted by therapists who wish to use treatments that work (Bohart, 2005; Glasziou, 2005; Lilienfeld, Ritschel, Lynn, Cautin, & Latzman, 2013).

## Basics

An ICF is a working hypothesis of how one client's problems are manifesting now and being maintained through patterns of cognition, emotional processing and behaviour. As classically described by Dudley, Kuyken, and Padesky (2011), Persons (1989) and Wells (1997), basic formulations will include an individual's strengths and vulnerability factors, as well as causal or triggering factors and also maintaining factors; the last of which are often part of the client's understandable response to threat or their own distress.

Working towards an integrated ICF assists in a clinician's assessment process. As the therapist takes a client history and conducts an assessment, naturally a lot of information is revealed. This is likely to take the form of historical detail about specific events, family structure and relationships, onset of problems, past efforts at fixing the problems and apparently unrelated issues. The CB therapist needs to learn to listen to and process all this information into something that is both manageable and useful. This then enables them to present it back to the client in a way that does several tasks simultaneously: (a) conveys that the therapist has been listening with interest, (b) helps the client form a self-compassionate view of what is happening to them, (c) reveals the key maintaining factors that could be disrupted, and thereby (d) generate a rationale for cognitive and behavioural interventions.

# Tips on developing helpful formulations

### 1. How to share the formulation with the client

Sharing the formulation needs to be done in a way that is mindful of how it might be received by each client. Some will become overwhelmed if the therapist tries to include everything that they noted in the assessment. The ICF and its discussion need to be collaborative, as with every step in cognitive therapy. It should be presented as a shared hypothesis — a 'live' document that you will both add to over time as you get to know the client and all the relevant factors better. After all, it is natural to deepen our collaborative understanding of the relevant factors after self-monitoring and early interventions reveal emotional, behavioural and cognitive details, and after the client learns to trust the therapist more over time.

Many therapists will try to share a brief formulation at the end of the first assessment consultation and this is commendable. The client will walk away feeling that things make sense and that there is new way to look for structured interventions. It provides contemplative clients with more information with which to make a decision about continuing with treatment. Early-career therapists are usually encouraged to take an extra consultation or two before presenting the ICF to their client, as this gives them time to discuss the assessment with a supervisor and give due consideration to the process. If the client needs extra care establishing the parameters of a safe and effective working relationship (e.g., with complex trauma or past negative therapy experiences), then it is unlikely that you will have achieved a sufficient assessment to have a useful ICF by the end of the first assessment consultation.

## 2. Know the theoretical models of a condition

The CBT literature includes several theoretical models of the cause and maintenance of certain diagnostic conditions. These are not the same as an ICF but it helps enormously to be familiar enough with these such that you are able to reproduce them. The main benefits of knowing published theoretical models include (a) using them as a guide for the assessment: knowing what vulnerability and maintaining factors to look out for, (b) enabling some psychoeducation and compassionate validation through the assessment (e.g., 'the desire to suppress your memories is understandable and actually research also tells us that it is one of the most common maintaining factor for other PTSD symptoms for many people'), and (c) helping to structure the layout of the initial ICF sketch, (e.g., the theoretical model might indicate how much space to leave for core beliefs and where the core beliefs might be best placed in relation to the main presenting symptom). Thus, knowing these theoretical formulations and models confers on the clinician both efficiency and confidence as they generate a formulation *de novo* for the client in front of them.

Another way to state this point is that it is highly desirable to know theoretical formulations, but we almost never share them in a session with a client. A client may not feel that they are being heard, treated as a unique individual or having their pain validated if the therapist resorts to a textbook or pre-printed formulation. The ICF is more memorable and relatable for a client if they see it emerge in front of them, using their language. The rare exceptions when a standardised (published) formulation sketch might be helpful include *bibliotherapy* (if you work with the same clinical population repeatedly, such as an anxiety disorders or chronic pain clinic) or if you were doing *group therapy* (in which case each client cannot readily have a personally tailored formulation).

An example of this might be Clark and Wells' model of social phobia (1995), which is very useful for understanding the condition, guiding assessment and providing a rationale for key treatment procedures (see Figure 2.1).

If we try to apply this model to Monica (our 21-year-old client with social anxiety), several key adaptations would be helpful as you can see in Figure 2.2. Firstly, rather than saying 'processing self as a social object',

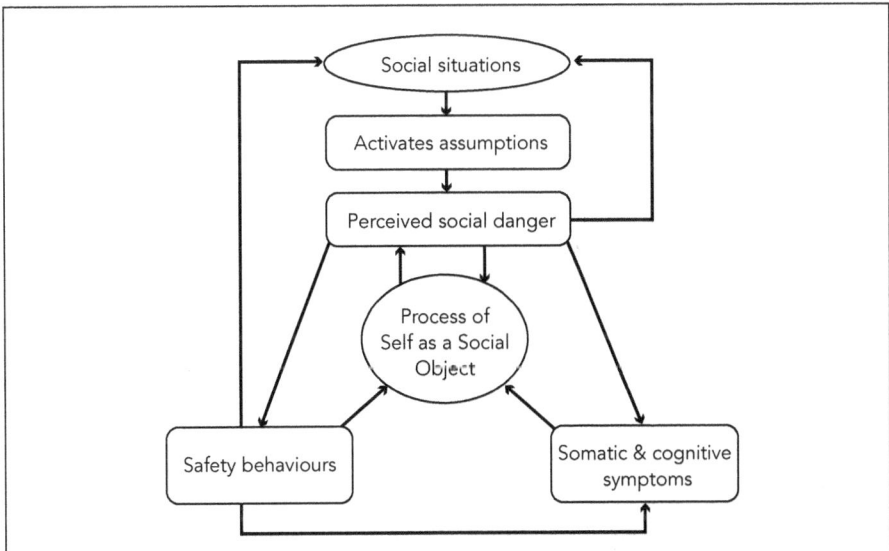

**FIGURE 2.1**
Clark and Wells' cognitive model of social anxiety.

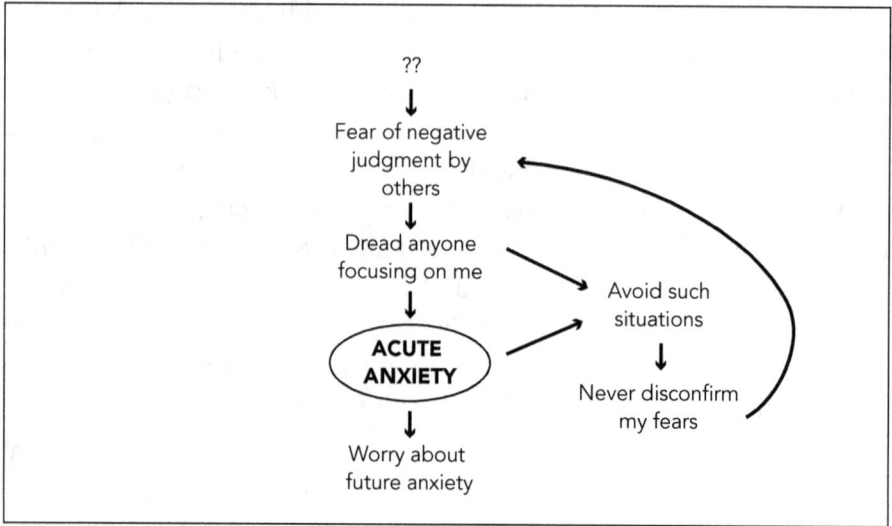

**FIGURE 2.2**
Monica — social anxiety, acute anxiety, worry and sleep disturbance.

which may confuse or alienate this client, use a phrase that she has used herself — perhaps 'dread anyone focusing on me'. Secondly, it may be profitable at some point to add her comorbid conditions of sleep disturbance, worry and what maintains her worry.

The therapist chooses to start with the phrases that Monica uses herself: 'anxiety', 'dread anyone focusing on me'. Monica is very aware of the avoidance, so this can be added to the ICF sketch immediately. The therapist chooses to add the avoidance in a way that helps therapist and client see how avoidance prevents the disconfirmation of the original fear. The therapist then chooses to add the element 'Fear of negative judgement by others' as an additional step, which helps them to collaborate on the task of accounting for the dread in certain situations. In Figure 2.2 (the start of her ICF), the question marks are left at this session because the assessment is yet to reveal why Monica is so much more fearful of evaluation than most people her age.

It takes quite a few sessions for the formulation to evolve to this level shown in Figure 2.3. Monica takes some time to trust her therapist with the idea that she feels safer being in a sick-role and the therapist needed a few more sessions to develop the hypothesis of maturity fears.

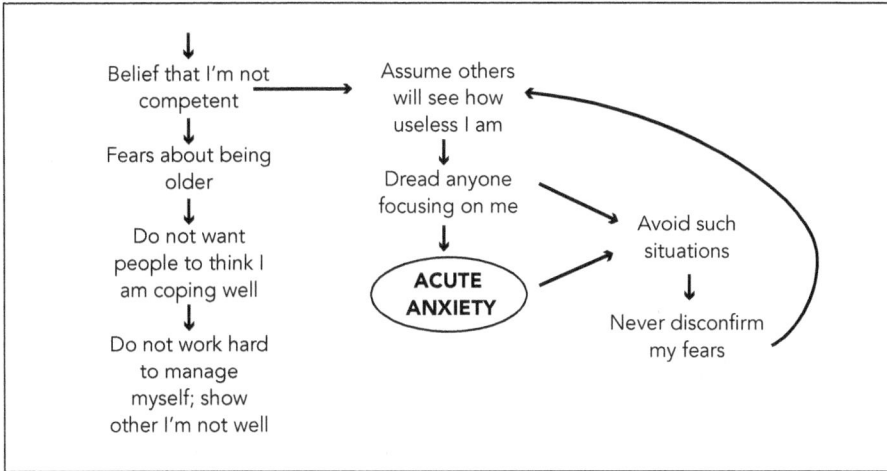

**FIGURE 2.3**
A more developed sketch of Monica's ICF.

Consider the strengths and weaknesses of this ICF sketch for Monica. It is individually tailored — using her own phrases, such as, 'I am not competent' but also note that this is clearly labelled as a belief, thus a target for cognitive intervention. It now makes more sense to Monica why she dreads anyone focusing on her. Her missing out on the opportunity to disprove the fear is our core rationale for starting some behavioural experiments soon and asking Monica how she can act differently to produce a happier future that is still safe.

Yet, what might be missing from this ICF? Might Monica feel that her problems are over-simplified? At this point, her problem with sleep has not been included and there is no mention of her other complaints like fear of talking in class at college or feeling 'completely screwed up'.

When at the point of sketching an ICF, attending to the alliance is crucial. It is reasonable to check-in with your client by asking what they think and feel about the content and arrangement of the formulation. It is equally reasonable to explain that this is just one part of your understanding for now and the degree of understanding will evolve and clarify over time. If there is poor agreement or any sign of negative affect, it pays to take the time to explore these responses before proceeding with the ICF.

Combining your knowledge of the generic published formulations with your assessment of your current client means the therapist can tailor each formulation to that individual. Examples of useful formulations from the literature include Clark's model of panic attacks (Clark, 1986), Barlowe and Craske's (2001) model of panic disorder, Treasure's cognitive interpersonal maintenance model of anorexia nervosa (Treasure & Schmidt, 2013), Wilson and Fairburn's formulation of bulimia nervosa (Fairburn, 2008), Clark's model of social phobia (Clark, 1995; Wells & Clark, 1997) or Salkovskis' model of obsessive anxiety (Salkovskis, Forrester, & Richards, 1998). In health psychology, it is extremely helpful to be familiar with a classic formulation of chronic pain (Vlaeyen & Linton, 2002), illness anxiety (Salkovskis, 1989; Warwick & Salkovskis, 1990) and panic attacks (Clark, 1986).

Another source of generic or 'nomothetical' formulations can be found in highly recommended texts such as Beck (1995), Persons (1989), or Persons and Tompkins (2007). These include standard components such as vulnerability factors, triggers, antecedent cognitions, symptoms, maintaining factors, individual strengths, and the like. These are also worth studying for familiarity but the strongest formulations will emerge in front of the client, with them as co-authors. Thus, the ICF becomes a tool of empathic listening as well as a clear rationale for individually tailored treatment. If the therapist uses a generic template then none of this can be achieved.

### 3. What medium?

Therapists have access to various methods and media for writing notes and sketching formulations within a consultation. Many continue to use blank paper that the client and therapist can keep copies of. A variation of this is for the client to purchase a notebook or folder in which all their monitoring and notes get recorded and compiled. Other therapists prefer the option of a whiteboard in the consulting room, while others have adopted various screen-based devices (e.g., tablets) and never use paper. There is no optimal medium for doing ICFs. The therapist can feel free to use whatever medium works well for their clients. Even if you prefer a paperless office, some (e.g., older) clients may still have a strong prefer-ence for a piece of paper to look at and refer back to. In this case, the paperless-office therapist would need to print a copy. The same goes with a whiteboard — a digital or paper copy needs to be retained so the client and therapist can keep referring to the sketch and accompanying notes.

Whatever medium is used, the ICF notes and sketch ought to meet several criteria: (a) it is user-friendly for that particular client, (b) the sketched diagram is visible to the client and is easily shared in session, (c) a permanent file copy can be retained for viewing each session, and (d) it can be altered or added to over time.

### 4. Where to start?
It can be hard to know where to begin when sketching or writing out a client's ICF. The most common starting point is whatever the client identifies as their major problem is. This is one of the many ways that a good ICF can aid the therapeutic relationship, as the client will sense that their therapist is attuned to their needs and is listening accurately to what they are saying. It may be the case that the therapist sees or believes that there is a higher-order presenting issue or perhaps can see a causal issue that needs addressing first in therapy. Nevertheless, it is still possible and desirable to start with what the client states is their primary concern that they want help with. The additional elements can be added with time.

This is illustrated in the cases of 'Amanda' and 'Neil', which we will examine very soon. We will also meet a new client for the first and last time: 'Frank'.

In the case of Amanda (our sample client with panic disorder), a good starting point may be the issues causing her the most distress — her fear that she will 'lose control', faint or collapse. This would be the first thing that is written down (with Amanda looking on, and the therapist checking with her that it seems accurate to her). Added next could be elements such as how bad her past anxiety has felt, allowing the therapist to make empathic and validating statements such as, 'it makes sense that you would want to avoid places where you can predict you would feel that bad'. The therapist may enquire if she tends to scan or check her body for signs of danger and then, at this point, add the vigilant monitoring as another element (see Figure 2.4).

The next step in sketching the ICF might be to add additional elements and arrows to highlight the self-maintaining power of the vigilance and

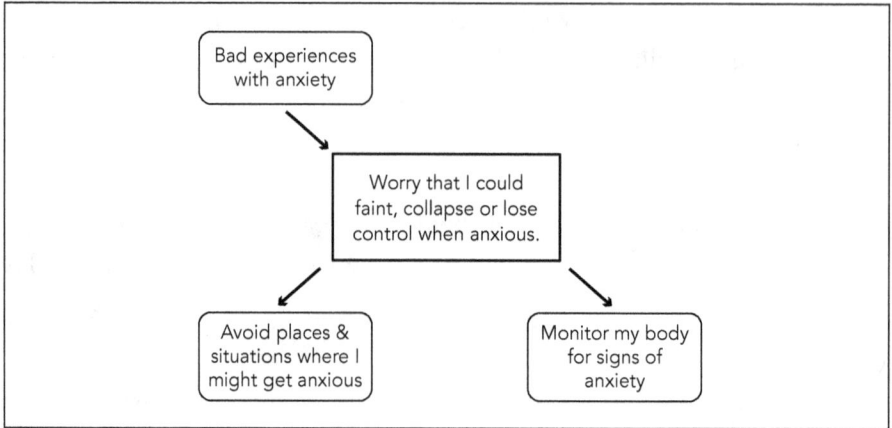

**FIGURE 2.4**
The starting sketch of Amanda's formulation (panic disorder).

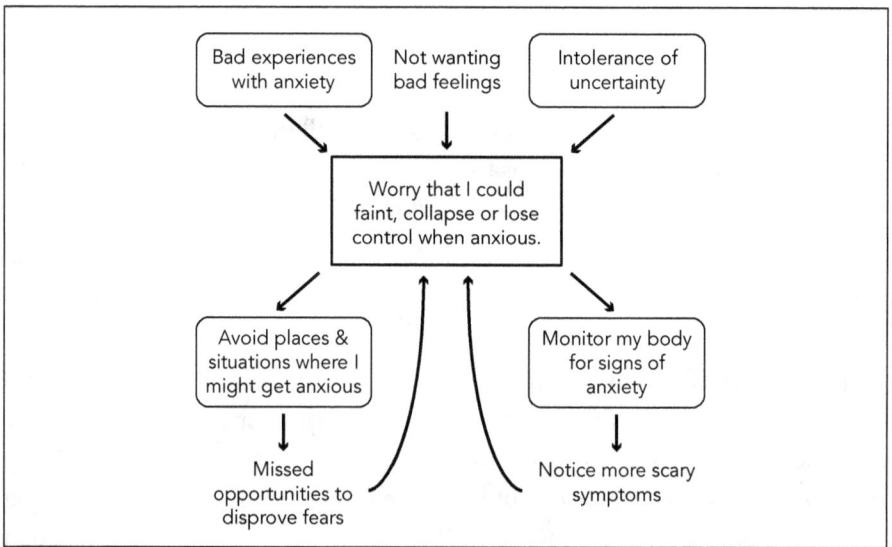

**FIGURE 2.5**
Macro-formulation of Amanda (panic disorder).

avoidance (see Figure 2.5). The therapist would most commonly add this in a process of psychoeducation. However, these elements could be elicited from the client through Socratic questioning before proceeding to explain (didactically) what they think is occuring. In the case of Amanda, the two extra elements of 'not wanting bad feelings' and 'intolerance of uncertainty' are added in the next consultation, as the therapeutic discussion continues to identify and explore these traits that she possesses. These elements do not necessarily apply to everyone and are not found in most generic theoretical models, but in this case the therapist and she agreed that there is evidence of their existence and influence.

If you are sketching the ICF, then where you position the first item (usually the presenting problem) depends on how well you can conceive the overall formulation. This is when a knowledge of nomothetic formulations and published theoretical models is very helpful. For instance, if you can see that a maladaptive schema is driving fear of negative evaluation in Monica's social phobia, a space would be left for that. Likewise, if you can anticipate some maintaining factors that would be best placed below the presenting issue on the page, a space would also be left for that.

Occasionally, the problem that the client declares to be the main problem may need careful reframing. Let's look at the example of Frank, a new sample client whom we have not yet met in this book.

Frank is a 77-year-old widower who lost his wife Anna three years ago to cancer. He is in a new relationship with Marie, a woman roughly his age, and they are thinking of marriage. The problem that he wants treatment for, he says, is 'pathological grief'. However, a thorough assessment suggests to the therapist that his level of sadness and his grieving process (thoughts, memories and behaviours) are well within the normal range. Imagine that you are the therapist. You are cautious not to invalidate him by refuting that this is his problem and yet, equally, you would not wish to collude with an unhelpful label or formulation. A way through this dilemma might be to write out what Frank says in a descriptive paraphrasing ('concern that my grief is excessive in severity or duration'). Then you and Frank can wonder together why he has the concern that this might be the case. This is illustrated in Figure 2.6.

Regarding his perception that his grief is not normal, Frank tells you that his new partner, Marie, has informed him that he has a problem with his pathological bereavement because of the way he still feels sad and talks about his wife. This enables a nonjudging explanation of his behaviours that Marie finds painfully challenging. For the record, these behaviours include Frank fondly recalling things that he and his wife did together or

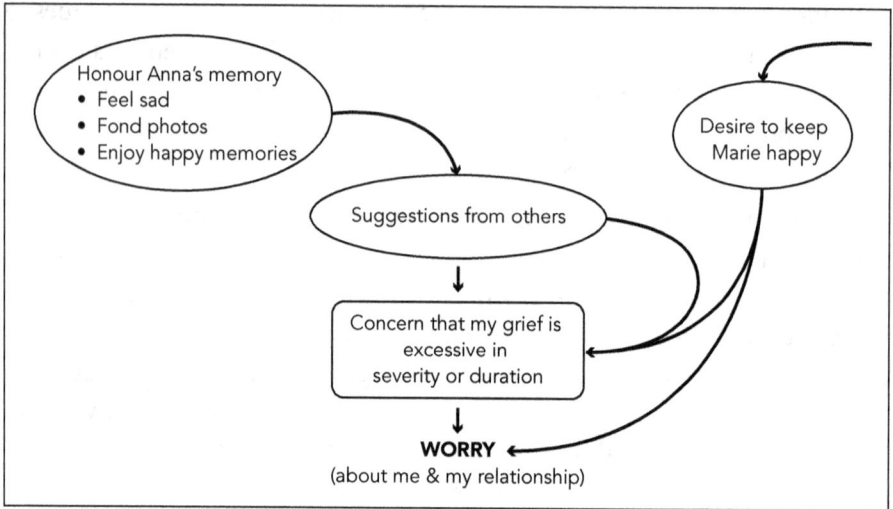

**FIGURE 2.6**
Sketched formulation of Frank: reframing a presenting issue misidentified by a client.

wanting to keep photos of her in the house, which he does to honour her memory and because it makes him feel good to recall their many happy years together. Marie says that these behaviours are a sign that he is struggling and is not over the grieving yet. She wants him to work on his feelings so that he is less sad and there is more room for their relationship to grow. Like all good ICFs, this formulation will hopefully make the recommended intervention evident to the client. In this case, it also permits you to do some education about grief. Then you and Frank can decide collaboratively how he can discuss things with Marie in a respectful and helpful way.

By inserting 'suggestions from others', Frank can see that he is placing a lot of importance on this. The therapist can respectfully differ in their opinion. The 'desire to keep Marie happy' needs to be articulated as natural and understandable. But the arrow above it highlights that at some point in therapy, it may help to explore just how important it is to Frank to keep his partner happy at all costs. The therapist is hypothesising that Frank may have internalised a self-sacrificing early maladaptive schema or perhaps he feels underserving or worthless and needs to work hard to have anybody accept him. An open arrow or a question mark can serve this purpose of alerting to an issue needing further enquiry in subsequent sessions.

## 5. Tailoring your formulation for purpose:

When sketching a diagrammatic formulation, the therapist ought to have at least one goal in mind. When the rationale for some (possibly difficult) treatment emerges from that formulation, then a client is likely to buy into that reasoning and hope, thus increasing their willingness to experiment with a step that they have never done. Depending on the stage of therapy and the nature of the problem, the primary goal may be any of the following: (a) psychoeducation, such as increasing a client's understanding of how various issues or factors are interlinked, (b) generating a shared rationale for treatment interventions, (c) increasing the client's willingness and their confidence that they can engage in these steps, and (d) as an aid to cognitive therapy, because a sketched diagrammatic formulation helps the 'decentring' or 'defusing' stance from emotion and familiar thoughts and beliefs. Another benefit (if not a 'goal') of an ICF sketch is to help keep the therapy process on track. This is discussed further in Chapter 7.

Optimal therapy is always intentional and purposeful and the clinician chooses to sequence treatments with strategic care. For instance, we cannot teach cognitive restructuring, problem-solving, assertiveness and behavioural activation all at the same time for a depressed client. As the therapist selects a part of the treatment to be prioritised, there may be one focal point for the psychoeducation and therefore the formulation. Thus, the clinician may need to highlight one particular aspect of the formulation over all others (indeed, at the temporary expense of other factors). This can and should be rectified a few sessions later when a new, additional formulation is developed with the client that highlights the other aspects of the whole formulation. Thus, a client is very likely to have more than one formulation sketch in their file notes.

Let's examine Amanda as an illustrative example again. When the clinician wishes to highlight the role of self-focused attention and misinterpreting benign physical symptoms in alarming ways, they might sketch a personalised version of Clark's cognitive model for her, shown in Figure 2.7

We have already seen one ICF sketch for Amanda (see Figure 2.5), which encompasses the way that her avoidance perpetuates her anxiety. When the therapeutic lens turns to the way she continues to worry (and doubt with obsessional quality) about her anxiety symptoms, the therapists draws a new sketch with her help, threading in the psychoeducation. You can no

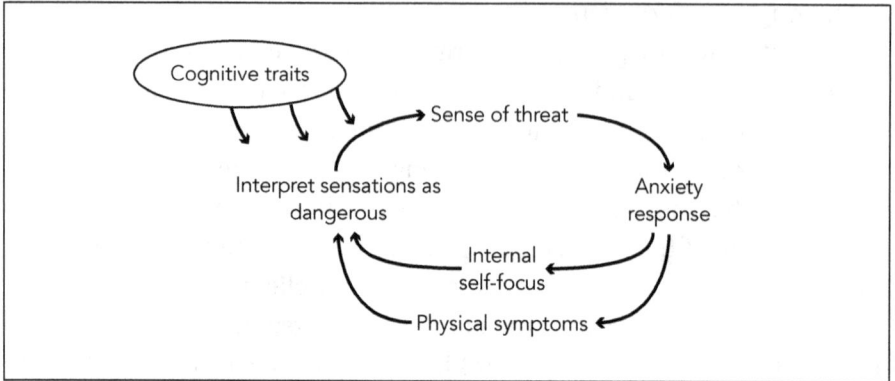

**FIGURE 2.7**
Micro-formulation of Amanda's panic attacks.

doubt see the educational points the therapist is trying to make. In this example (see Figure 2.7), one key issue is the role of vigilant monitoring of her physical symptoms while the other is the misinterpretation of benign physical states. And what cognitive therapy skills and interventions seem to emerge as potentially helpful from this diagram?

In the same sketch, the 'cognitive traits' are alluded to but not in any detail; these will be expanded in a new focused ICF sketch highlighting her thinking patterns that make her vulnerable to misinterpretation of benign sensations and vigilant body-scanning.

In the next example (see Figure 2.8), the therapist here is hoping to teach *tolerating uncertainty* and *defusing from emotion* (especially her sense of 'not-quite-right') and cognition ('you never quite know for sure'). Therefore, some different elements are included, including the cognitive trait of intolerance of uncertainty and how this interacts with the occurrence of physical sensations. You will also note the inclusion of some psychoeducation at this point, so the therapist is unilaterally authoring this aspect of the sketch (it is a purposeful treatment-oriented formulation diagram). Hopefully, Amanda will see (in a fresh, decentred way) the origin of her worry-thoughts and will be more likely to have helpful beliefs, such as giving herself permission to ignore or dispute those worry-thoughts.

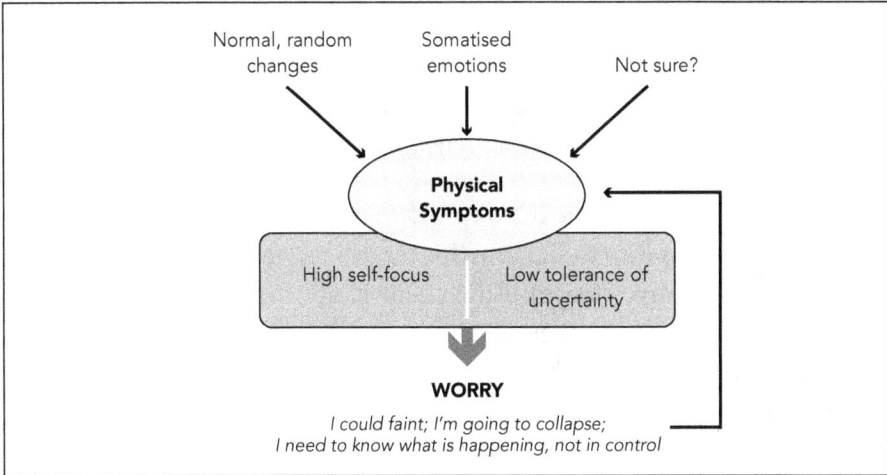

**FIGURE 2.8**
Amanda, with a particular therapeutic focus.

*6. Make sure that you are entirely on the same page as your client.*
For a start, you will be on the same page if the client feels that they have co-authored the formulation. Beck famously subtitled cognitive therapy as 'collaborative empiricism', and this collaborative stance starts with the formulation. When the therapy process becomes anything other than collaborative (for instance, when the therapist finds themselves working harder than the client or setting an agenda without a clear rationale for the client), then we slip towards therapeutic impotence. To achieve this, the therapist can ask their client, 'how would I word this?', or 'when you choose not to attend the dinner with friends, we know that fear causes this, but what are the consequences of that choice?', then 'shall I draw that in here or there?', and 'is this arrow one-way or bidirectional?'.

We can also pose certain questions to the client to the check the comprehension, effectiveness and utility of the formulation as we have it:

*Does it look like I've got it? Am I on the right track in understanding what is really happening for you?*

*What does this help to explain?*

*What might be missing — what does this not explain?*

23

> *So, does this help your understanding of what is going on? In what way?*
>
> *What does this sketch imply in terms of what problem we should work on first and also how we might do that?*

In this way, we can avoid the ICF being *delivered* or *pronounced* by the therapist-as-expert. It is easy to slip into this mode (and therefore away from the desirable collaborative stance) if the client is not forthcoming with information. In such cases, the therapist needs to take time to use the data from the client's experiences. This may come from prospective monitoring between sessions by asking for recent examples of symptom exacerbation.

As Leahy (2006; 2008) has powerfully explained, when the therapist and client have divergent theories about the nature of emotions, the reason they feel the way they do, or how to fix the problem, then types of resistance emerge. The case formulation is an important therapeutic method to discover if there are divergent ideas and develop a unified theory with your client.

A quick way to ensure that the clinician and client are on the same track can be done as you work on developing the formulation. Leahy has suggested the following four crucial questions in which there *must* be congruence before treatment can proceed:

1.  What is the nature of the problem?

2.  What are the contributing factors (causal and maintaining factors)?

3.  What treatment is most likely to work, given what we know about the problem?

4.  Whose responsibility is it to do that treatment?

### 7. Be willing and ready to modify your case formulation

It is inevitable that you will learn more about a client the longer you treat them, so the formulation often evolves. There are many reasons why the best of therapists cannot know everything about their client at the end of the third session: the client may lack insight; they are not sure what is relevant; they may not be sure they can yet trust you with everything; a new situation sheds fresh light on the presenting issue; their coping strategies are all based on emotional avoidance, which prevents access to key material; and so on. Therefore, we actually *want* to modify the formulation over time, rather than protect one formed at a certain point in time.

For other clients, a revolution is required more than evolution. When Neil reveals more about his personal history, it changes everything. When his wife provides data about his drinking, it changes again. Monique's therapist needs a few sessions to realise the pervasive pattern of avoidance and the core fear of people seeing how incompetent she is. This provokes a substantial change in the formulation from anxiety to personality disorder.

It is easy to become anxious or feel completely wrong-footed when personal information arises that is inconsistent with your current formulation. We do well when we remind ourselves and our clients that every case formulation is a hypothesis that needs to be refined — and that every change is an advancement, not an admission of error. Indeed, Needleman (2006) advises therapists to try to seek out evidence that is inconsistent with the extant formulation. This is perhaps the only way to avoid a confirmation bias process. The ICF will be more accurate and helpful to the client if they and the therapist are willing to challenge it and let it evolve with more data over time.

## 8. Managing comorbidity in an ICF

When the client has more than one condition (and we know that comorbidity is the general *rule*, not the *exception*), then the clinician has a few options. It might make sense to do a formulation centred around just one of the symptoms or one of the diagnoses. This choice would make sense if you wished to start the treatment with one condition prioritised over the other (for reasons of safety or client preference) or to assist psychoeducation for the client, focused on one issue at a time, which assists in the learning of new material.

The other alternative is to generate and sketch a formulation which combines several overlapping issues. This is especially helpful if the client is yet to see the link between the issues or if their motivation to address one problematic behaviour is low but that behaviour is a maintaining factor for one of the conditions. For example, a client wants help with depression. They say that their marijuana use is one of the few things that they enjoy in life and they list it as a pleasant event to help them pull out of the depression. The therapist can try to include exactly what the client says into the formulation and, with time and evidence, introduce the idea that the cannabis may be having some negatives alongside the perceived benefits (such as financial expense, impact on relationships, reduced motivation, reduced time to do other activities, reduced productivity, increased anxiety, and so on).

Let us take a final look at the ICF for Monica, who initially came with social anxiety. After some discussion, she and her therapist realised that there were deeper concerns along the lines of Avoidant Personality Disorder, with a fear of being found to be incompetent, and this was manifesting as a fear of maturity. She also was distressed by her sleep-onset insomnia. By way of reminder, the ICF achieved by session four was the one shown already in Figure 2.3.

Here is how the therapist expands her ICF sketch to make sense of the additional elements of worry and sleep disturbance. First, the therapist highlights the fundamental causal relationship between low tolerance of uncertainty and worry. Monica is not necessarily aware of this, but the therapist is aware of the theory about this and, after some brief psychoeducation and the checking in with her, Monica agrees that (a) she feels very uncomfortable with uncertainty and goes to lengths to avoid it, (b) this leads her to have positive metacognitions about worry — beliefs that worry helps her to be safe and solve problems and (c) that this then increases the time that she engages in worry-type thoughts. Figure 2.9 shows how the therapist chose to write this in. Note that Monica and the therapist make a link between the worrying at night and the trouble with sleep onset. This is based on a brief examination of Monica's prospective monitoring and a retrospective assessment ('Tell me about the last two nights that you had trouble sleeping, can you recall if you were worrying about things?').

The therapist makes the connection that it makes sense to fear growing older if Monica truly believes that she is not competent to be in the world on her own. A further connection made here is that that the combined influence of intolerance of both mistakes and uncertainty has contributed to her sense of incompetence is. If Monica *needs* to feel *sure* that she will never make a mistake, then she is frozen — unable to take action. Thus, all the elements seem to make sense and can be represented in the one diagram.

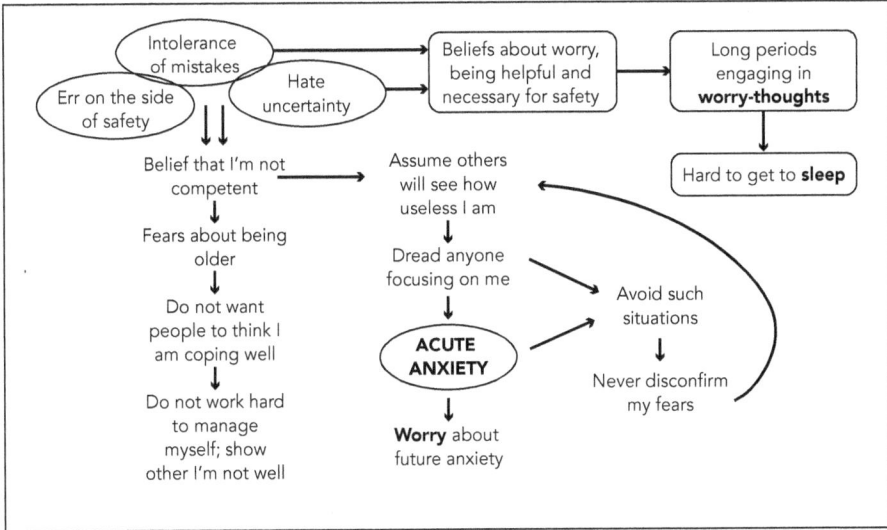

**FIGURE 2.9**
Extended ICF sketch of Monica's multiple resenting issues.

This leaves Monica with the clear rationale that she can work on her stable cognitive traits of (a) not tolerating uncertainty, (b) rules about the impermissibility of mistakes — a virulent feature of unhealthy perfectionism, and (c) her metacognitions about worry. In the future, if she says she really needs to work on her sleep, then the therapist might spend some time on sleep hygiene or relaxation but will devote much more time to metacognitive therapy for worry, as this is the main driver of the problem.

### 9. An example of an evolving set of ICFs for the one client.
Looking at Neil's formulation (our client with depression) is illustrative of several instructional points raised thus far in this chapter. The two sketches following (see Figure 2.10 and Figure 2.11) demonstrate that it helps to have varying formulations at different points and to serve a range of purposes. And this can be done in a way that uses the client's own words and shows compassion for their struggles. In Neil's case, starting with a simple sketch of the factors contributing to his depression, in which the chief purpose is to provide a rationale for using cognitive therapy skills (by introducing Beck's depressive cognitive triad of the self, world and future) and behavioural activation (because the depressive symptoms such as

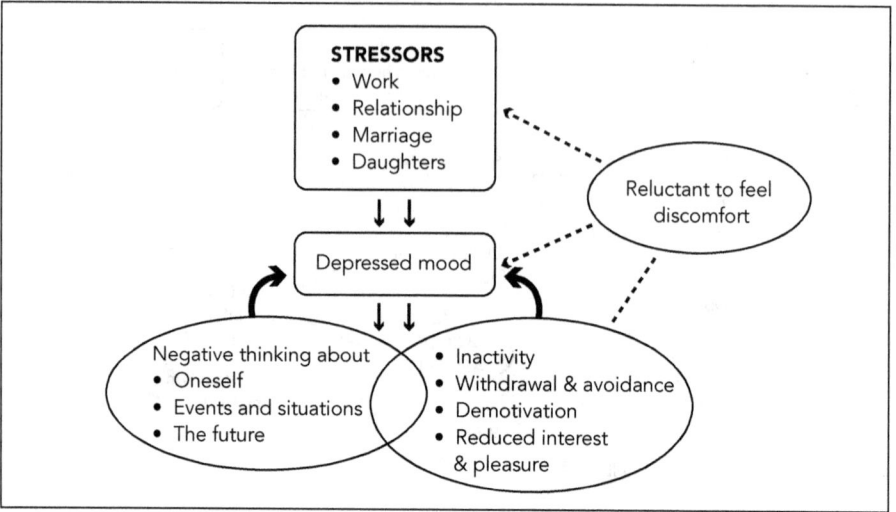

**FIGURE 2.10**
Neil's initial ICF sketch.

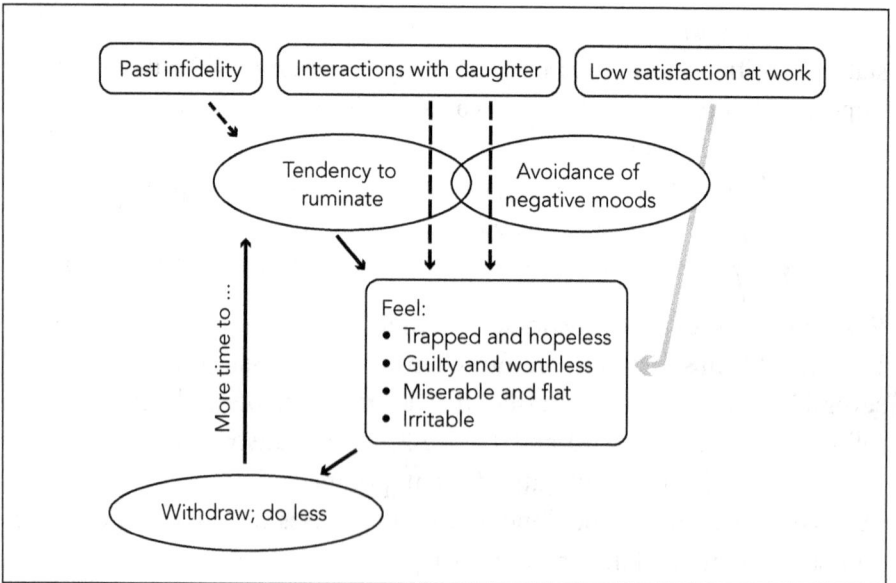

**FIGURE 2.11**
Neil's ICF with a focus on cognitive processing style.

demotivation and social withdrawal can beget further depression if a person acts on them).

Note the choice to include 'reluctant to feel discomfort'. To avoid conveying any judgement — the therapist can normalise this with statements such as:

*No human naturally likes discomfort.*

*We all recoil away from physical pain.*

*Emotional pain is no different.*

*We all have many small, habitual ways that we minimise emotional discomfort.*

*It makes sense for us to examine the various ways the you might do this because the extent to which we can tolerate discomfort has a huge impact on our ability to fight depression and then maintain emotional health.*

Actually, the therapist hypothesises that Neil's willingness and capacity to tolerate emotional pain is very low, especially with certain emotions and especially with his daughter but chooses to address this slowly over a few more sessions, allowing for the therapeutic alliance (TA) to strengthen and for Neil to establish insight at a pace tolerable to Neil.

The next formulation sketch for Neil highlights these elements more directly. Neil has said that he feels hopeless about getting better because he has so many issues keeping him miserable: he hates his work but cannot leave, he hates himself for the affair and refuses to tell his wife, and he feels bound up in a relationship with his daughter who is very unhappy and seems to need all his resources. Neil also says that his thinking is not the problem — these three problems are 'real' and are causing his depression. So, the therapist tries to acknowledge what Neil is saying by using his words and writing the three problems into the sketch (top level). The therapist adds a second level of cognitive *processing* (which is as important in cognitive therapy as cognitive *content*). These are a tendency for ruminating on past events and emotional avoidance, seen on the second level of Figure 2.11. This level is designed to provide a rationale for doing some cognitive therapy work, given that it is now clear that Neil's thinking about the stressors can be the focus of intervention more than the stressors themselves. The target of the cognitive therapy can go beyond what he thinks, to encompass how often and how long he thinks it.

There is a direct line from low work satisfaction to depressive feelings to help acknowledge what Neil says. There are dotted lines from the other two stressors and these are deliberately drawn to go through the filtering effect of the cognitive processing styles. This is designed to highlight that the thinking and emotional processing is important. In the bottom corner is a reference to the well-known link between depressive symptoms of inactivity leading to even more ruminating, which in turn leads to more depressed affect.

This ICF sketch sits in a visible space in the consulting room for the next several sessions as a conscious reminder to Neil and the therapist that there is cognitive therapy work to be done on the stressors, as opposed to simple problem-solving, for Neil's pessimism.

### 10. Some final notes

Certain exercises can be helpful for the therapist who wishes to enhance their formulation skills, including practicing with every client, drawing out more than one formulation per client, take your formulations to supervision discussions, and look at and learn from others. An additional exercise is to sketch ICF's from a novel perspective such as addressing this question for a client's point of view: 'why I am stuck and cannot get better on my own?'.

Non-typical factors to consider including in your formulation include:

- Relational patterns or attachment style (see Chapter 3)

- Motivational balance for change and therapy (see Chapter 4)

- Cognitive style and personal recurring biases (see Chapter 5)

- Schemas (see Chapter 5).

Invest time in developing good case formulation skills that are individually tailored because a flexible formulation if often your best tool in preventing and responding to challenges and roadblocks in therapy (Leahy, 2006; Tompkins, 1999).

# Highlights and take-home messages

1.  An ICF that encompasses the key clinical data about a client can help the clinician manage the most common obstacles and challenges that arise in therapy.

2.  Become familiar with published theoretical models for common diagnosable conditions, as these will help you to look out for the causal and maintaining factors in your assessment and will help you arrange your thinking and ICF.

3.  Each ICF should be tailored to the individual and should be centred around helping explain the rationale for the treatment that makes the most sense

4.  A good formulation sketch will assist with psychoeducation and will deepen the therapeutic relationship.

# Chapter 3

# Developing, managing and using the therapeutic relationship

A technique-oriented approach to CB practice that minimises or trivialises the importance of the therapeutic alliance is likely to lead to poor client compliance and a high drop-out rate.

(Grant, Mills, Mulhern, & Short, 2004)

I t is a truth universally acknowledged that the therapeutic alliance (TA) is important for psychological therapy. Furthermore, most clinicians think or assume that we are quite skilled at building rapport. Yet, do we check that our skills in this regard are sufficient for each client and achieving the outcomes that we want? Is the TA on our minds as much as it ought to be each session? Are we willing to find out how our clients rate the TA with us?

## What is the therapeutic relationship and alliance?

The terms 'therapeutic relationship', 'therapeutic alliance', 'helping alliance' and 'working alliance' are often used interchangeably. Some argue with good reason that the therapeutic *relationship* is broader than the *alliance*, which is one of its essential constituent parts. This chapter focuses on the TA, as it has received the most focus in terms of research evidence and documentation of the skills that therapists can develop to improve it.

Many still turn to Bordin's (1979) early analysis of the chief constituent parts of the TA: (1) the quality of the emotional bond, which is the extent to which the client feels understood, accepted and respected; (2) the degree of collaboration between the therapist and client on agreed therapeutic tasks; and (3) their shared view of the desired outcomes or goals.

Much of this book is devoted to encouraging therapists to do the technical cognitive and behavioural interventions in highly accurate ways, as this will help get results. However, it would be a grave reduction of CBT to consider it purely a technique-driven mode of treatment. There is evidence that no matter how behavioural the treatment must ultimately be, our clients respond to our interactions with emotions and opinions. The same broad body of research reminds us that there are patterns in how people respond to the therapy and their therapist — that every person seeking emotional help comes with their own set of attachment style, their own emotional history of being treated a certain way, their own beliefs and expectations about emotions and healing. We select a treatment because we have reason to believe it will work. Yet, each treatment program with proven effectiveness in a trial must still be administered from one human to another.

It is right to think about the technical details of therapy and how best to teach our clients how to get better. The technical and the interpersonal aspects of therapy support each other. Wright and Davis (1994, p. 27) take Bordin's (1979) three key ideas and highlight the circular interdependence of the strategic training we do as CB therapists and the alliance with our clients: 'The bond affects the degree of agreement and this in turn affects the quality of the emotional bond. Thus, technical and relationship factors are interdependent parts within a single process in psychotherapy ... interpersonal interaction is the context in which techniques gain meaning and effectiveness'.

# How important is the TA and relationship?

The nonspecific elements of psychological therapy have been declared to account for considerable proportions of treatment outcomes (Safran & Muran, 2000; Wampold, 2001) even when comparing directive, strategic treatments like CBT to supportive psychotherapy (Arnow et al., 2013). Moreover, in line with the main thrust of this book, the more challenging the constellation of presenting problems, the more the therapist relies on the therapeutic relationship to achieve desired outcomes. For instance, those with a history of complex trauma are bound to have attachment disturbances that will play out in the therapeutic relationship (Freeman, 1992; Leahy, 2006; Liotti, 1991). Minor tremors of interpersonal insecurity need to be managed explicitly before the inevitable rupturing earthquake, such as when the clinician needs time off for illness or vacation or if the client detects frustration or boredom in their therapist. What is more, clients who have acquired negative schemas about themselves and others and those who have the greatest needs often require therapy that is more heavily reliant on the working relationship (Freeman, 1992; Leahy, 2006; Needleman, 2006). It is well established that one powerful way to repair and replace a core belief of worthless defectiveness is through the therapeutic relationship (Kazantzis, Dattilio & Dobson, 2017; Leahy, 2006; Liotti, 1991; Young, Klosko, & Weishaar, 2003).

In his thorough and repeated examination of psychotherapy outcome studies, Wampold concluded that, regardless of the treatment approach used, some therapists consistently achieve better outcomes than others (Wampold, 2006). For example, while IPT and CBT were found on average to be equally effective for depression, some IPT and some CBT clinicians consistently achieved better results, even though all were experienced and fully qualified and adhered to the treatment manual of that study (Kim, Wampold, & Bolt, 2006). A remarkable demonstration of this effect was witnessed when it was found that more effective psychiatrists, meeting regularly with patients, achieve better outcomes administering a placebo than do less effective psychiatrists administering antidepressant medication (McKay, Imel, & Wampold, 2006).

In one of the earliest descriptions of CBT, Beck, Rush, Shaw, and Emery (1979) reminded therapists that the therapeutic characteristics of warmth, genuineness and accurate empathy are *necessary* for positive change in therapy. Beck's thesis, though, and the basis for CBT is that such characteristics on their own are usually not *sufficient* to produce change when treating psychopathology; it is the procedural work, done with technical skill in a sufficient dose that is also necessary. To go further, it is well argued that therapists who rely alone on the therapeutic relationship for change are either arrogantly misguided (Freeman & McCloskey, 2006) or ignorantly underusing treatments that do work (Waller & Turner, 2016).

Treatment outcomes are influenced by many factors and much is understood about the variables that the clinician is able to control and these are highlighted in this chapter. The key aspects of the therapy relationship that have been well studied and summarised here are (1) a clinically potent TA that is strengthened through the clinician's expression of warmth and positive regard, empathy and validation; (2) noticing and managing ruptures in the relationship and (3) managing 'resistance' in its different forms. This chapter offers guidelines for improving clinicians existing skills in responding to clients in a way that makes each person seeking help feel more inclined to work hard in therapy and engage in the collaborative empiricism that becomes effective treatment.

## Therapist qualities and skills that deepen the bond and therapeutic alliance

The following list offers a summary of several key authors who have contributed to these guidelines. Firstly, Wright and Davis (1994) have listed several micro-skills and other qualities that a therapist needs to possess and use repeatedly and consciously to promote a TA. Wampold and colleagues (Baldwin, Wampold, & Imel, 2007; Duncan, Miller, Hubble, & Wampold, 2010; Miller, Hubble & Duncan, 2007; Wampold, 2007) have shared data on what variables seem to make some therapists better than others, including what they have termed 'supershrinks' the clinicians who reliably get better results than their equally trained peers. To the literature, Leahy has added excellent depth of understanding on factors that contribute to a deeper TA (Leahy, 2008) as well as client and therapist factors that can potentially detract from a good alliance, with advice on how to manage such risk factors (Leahy, 2006). Safran has consistently contributed important research and clinical recommendations for many years (Safran, 1998; Safran & Muran, 2000; Safran, Muran, Samstag & Stevens, 2002; Safran & Segal, 1990). Johns, Barkham, Kellett, and Saxon (2018, p. 90) have added to the literature on 'therapist effects' in treatment outcomes in a review of 20 studies, concluding that their review 'therapists make an important contribution to the variability in patient outcomes … with larger effects occurring with more severe patients'. Some of the better therapists in the studies they examined consistently produced results twice as good as colleagues within their own service. Their conclusions about helpful therapist qualities included mindfulness as therapist, time dedicated to improving therapy skills, ability to address avoidance in the client, ability to build a strong alliance, and possessing a flexible interpersonal style (Johns et al., 2018).

The following list comprises a compilation of the recommendations from all the authors cited above, through the prism of the clinical experience of the current author.

### Conscious work on the therapeutic relationship

- Assume responsibility for the alliance and rapport. That responsibility does not lie with the client, although they often do contribute to the relationship and many clients are easy to like. Those needing the most therapeutic help may be the least likely to be warm and trusting in the first several appointments. Not only will some clients not be invested in developing a good working alliance, their past experiences of rejection and humiliation may require them to operate strong defences of distrust and distancing with little or no insight. It is the therapist's responsibility to notice their own feelings and manage the relationship.

- Raise the topic of the working relationship as soon as appropriate. This may be alluded to in early psychoeducation or talked about at greater length when a more complex client is struggling. Raising this topic (e.g., talking about trust, attunement, validation, their feelings) is also the therapist's responsibility; and doing so signals to the client that you consider the working alliance important and are comfortable discussing it.

- Ensure that the treatment environment is warm and comfortable, yet professional, where a sense of safety is prioritised. Be alert to the inevitable 'house-blindness' — when we no longer notice elements in the treating environment that are unprofessional, distracting or uncomfortable.

## Convey warmth and a positive regard

- Create and use opportunities to express a positive regard for the client. This could be through the enthusiasm that they see when you greet them at the start of follow-up appointments. It could be through clear positive statements when an occasion arises (which it will if you are looking for it). Positive regard could be conveyed through praise for effort and tolerating hard issues or through your constant effort to do the best for them and fight for the best outcome for them.

- A self-aware therapist will notice when they are not conveying warmth or positive regard and have some curiosity about any hesitation that they might have within a session (e.g., being 'busy' with session-planning or juggling different hypotheses, not realising how hard a task was for this client, fear of sounding too insincere).

## Core listening skills

- Use a complex range of attuned micro-skills in listening and responding to the client. The verbal micro-skills include reflective listening, deeper levels of validation (e.g., reflecting back more complex emotions and helping to make links), being perceptive enough then to empathise with the client's key emotions while still expressing warmth and acceptance.

- The nonverbal micro-skills include posture and facial expression, which can convey what is needed in that moment depending on what you are hearing. For instance, appropriate eye-contact is essential for a client to feel that you are listening and your facial affect needs to reflect the emotive content of what they disclose. There is evidence that slightly raised eyebrows help convey openness and friendliness, which may occasionally help clients who feel threatened or insecure.

## Be directive and stay on task

- Having time to listen is important but a good therapist will also set and stick to an agenda — the client does not want to feel that you are a pushover or that they are left uncontained or undirected. The early use of interpersonal warmth and sound micro-skills mean that you can interrupt and redirect appropriately when that is later required.

- Likewise, setting homework exercises and striving for emotional and behavioural changes early in therapy can be amongst the most powerful bonding events for clients. There is nothing like some early gains to make the client believe in you and the therapy.

- When you do set monitoring or homework, give it due attention in terms of time at the beginning of the next consultation. The homework is also a golden opportunity to offer praise (e.g., for effort) or to discuss why they did not complete it as discussed. If not done as planned, this also represents an opportunity to express acceptance of them as a person and your positive regard for them independent of action or compliance. (See Chapter 5 for a discussion on how to use motivational interviewing approaches to increase homework compliance).

## Alignment of beliefs

- The client needs to believe in the therapy process, so a therapist must be convincing in order to instil trust and hope in the treatment. This can occur when developing the individual case formulation (ICF) as well as at the phase of psychoeducation and then presenting a rationale for treatment.

- A good therapist will be alert to discrepancies between the client and therapist, especially in terms of expectations and beliefs about therapy and emotional change. Once detected, any such discrepancy will need to be discussed until some compromising alignment is achieved.

- Explicit agreement (between client and therapist) needs to be achieved quite early in the therapy process regarding the nature of the problem, how it can be treated (the mechanism of change) and where the responsibility for that change lies. This is a sine qua non of effective therapy.

### Flexibility in interpersonal style

- A good therapist will be flexible enough to adapt their communication to clients of different cultural and religious backgrounds. If your client is wedded to one way of thinking, then this might need to be integrated into your ICF and treatment process.

- Likewise, be flexible with communication and the pace of treatment to accommodate different levels of school education, socioeconomic status, gender or sexual orientation and the like.

- Find the right balance of personable warmth and approachability, with respectful observation of the person (being neither too casual nor familiar). Be willing to have a range of warmth and closeness in communicative style so that it is responsive to the client of a certain age, gender or cultural background.

### Monitoring and willingness to change

- Check in with the client often. Discuss if they hesitate or appear uncomfortable with an approach, even if they agree. The client must never feel *coerced* into any treatment.

- Regular (e.g., every appointment) monitoring of the therapy progress and change over time; being alert for lack of response to treatment or any deterioration. Examine what the obstacles to change might be, careful not to appear judgemental or critical of the client, and be willing to intensify treatment and discuss alternatives with the client. Consider using a short assessment tool every session, such as the Outcome Rating Scales (see further notes on this in the next section).

- Regular (e.g., every appointment) monitoring of the therapeutic alliance. Consider using a short assessment tool every session, such as the Session Rating Scale (see notes below).

### Managing ruptures

- If there are any ruptures of the therapeutic alliance (big or small), pause whatever you were working on or discussing and address what just occurred. Try to name what you observed and invite the client to talk about their feelings and where these come from. Let them know that you invite and feel comfortable with honest feedback and that this is an integral part of productive therapy (further discussion is provided later this chapter).

- Look for opportunities to generalise any strong emotional reactions or forms of resistance that the client has from one moment in therapy to other relationships and other day-to-day situations.

- Be able to monitor your own emotional responses within the consultation and manage these in order to remain client-focused, attentive and nonjudging. When regarded properly, therapist emotions in response to a client or therapy are a wonderful source of information about that client and the work that needs to be done.

### Use the alliance once it is developed

- Be willing to say out aloud what is happening but what is not yet articulated. This could be incongruence between client statement and their affect; or when you sense the client needs to adhere to the role of victim without being willing to think or act adaptively; or when their need for validation means that the therapy constantly halts as soon as change-oriented interventions are introduced; or the client has not done the homework for a third consecutive session and there must be an understandable reason for that. The ICF is a valuable tool for such communication.

- A strong alliance and trust in the process also means that the therapist can invite the client to do therapy exercises that might be a modest degree harder than they feel ready to do. Similarly, a therapist at times needs to set strong or even non-negotiable limits around the therapy (such as with self-harming behaviours, weight loss or therapy-interfering behaviours) and this is more likely to proceed well when the client is invested in the therapy relationship.

### Therapist qualities as behaviours

- The client perceives an effective therapist as 'natural' and 'real' — so show a little *real-self* in the way you talk. It is possible to retain a highly professional stance with appropriate boundaries, while still treating the client like they are a real person (not just-another-client). The conversational style that serves this goal might feel like you are talking with someone at work whom you like and admire (reasonably formal yet able to sound conversational; never patronising; respectful of their intelligence; showing a natural warmth; that person would feel that you are interested in them).

- Self-disclosure, though, is usually best kept to a minimum. Before sharing information about oneself, there must be a very clear way in which this information will aid treatment and you must be very confident that the client will not start to think about your issues. Even sharing a commonality (such as both the client and therapist have two teenagers) needs to be done thoughtfully, in case the client then engages in unhelpful (e.g., self-critical or competitive) comparisons.

- Use humour judiciously. If it is appropriate, some occasional humour can advance the bond between therapist and client through demonstrating that you have a positive regard and that some levity is welcome amidst a very serious discussion. On the other hand, humour can dilute a desired sense of gravity (e.g., when discussing safety or urgency) and some clients may find it invalidating.

- Be a good example through modelling self-care and pacing; demonstrate how to meet one's own needs. Similarly, manage your own issues to prevent the client being focused on you.

It might be worth considering what *you* would be willing to do in order to move towards the rank of a 'supershrink'. Would you:

- Record (sound or video) your consultations and review them regularly with or without a supervisor to get clearer feedback on your micro-skills and attunement?

- Ask your clients for feedback at the end of each session?

- Reflect within supervision which clients you find it easier to express warmth and positive regard towards and with whom do you find this hard?

- Doing a behavioural experiment of your own to test out slightly new ways to interact with greater authenticity?

- What else came to mind about self-development as a therapist as you read this chapter?

A final note of encouragement: just when you think the bond with your client strong is healthy and productive, then it is time to keep attending to it:

> It is important to think of the therapeutic alliance as an ongoing process, rather than an achievement that is fixed at one point in time, since the relationship is interactive and iterative, reflecting the patient's response to the therapist's response to the patient'. (Leahy, 2008)

## Ways to monitor and measure the strength of your TA

Several studies powerfully remind the therapist not to rely on your own perception of the TA — we need to ask our client their views on the alliance. In their meta-analysis of 24 studies Horvarth and Symonds (1991) found that TA was highly predictive of treatment response but that the ratings of the TA by the clients was more predictive than clinician or observer ratings of the strength of the TA.

Several tools exist to assess help the clinician reliably monitor the TA, including the Penn Helping Alliance Scales (Alexander & Luborsky, 1986) and the Working Alliance Scale (Horvath & Greenberg, 1989), which are both relatively long and more often used in research than daily clinical work. The scales developed and disseminated by Miller and Duncan's team provide a briefer and useful alternative. The Outcome Rating Scales (Miller, Duncan, Brown, Sparks, & Claud (2003) are designed to monitor the client's ratings of improvement on four items (personal wellbeing, close relationships, work and social activity). It is designed to be given at the start of every session and the results charted and shared. The Session Rating Scale (Duncan, Miller, Sparks, Claud, Reynolds, Brown & Johnson, 2003) is designed to measure the client's experience of therapeutic alliance. It is administered at the end of very session and results are immediately discussed. One idea behind this is that the therapist would alter treatment to increase ratings so that the client experiences treatment as more helpful. Another possibility is that a lower rating could trigger a discussion about expectations and beliefs about the nature if the problem and what treatment is required. The therapist–client alignment of such beliefs has already been highlighted as essential for effective therapy.

A more fundamental idea is that the therapist knows when the client is feeling that the alliance is weaker and can attend to this, while at the same time signalling that that it is acceptable and helpful to discuss negative feelings about this important professional relationship. Furthermore, whenever you study something, that observation usually changes it. Studying and measuring the TA alerts both the client and therapist to the process in a way that is usually helpful. Not all clients will need or benefit from the repeated use of these tools but it is worth considering and trialling in most clinical settings.

In the case study of Amanda (panic attacks) a regular monitoring of the alliance and of the progress of therapy would enable her and the therapist to discuss the plateauing of changes early in the process — possibly saving a few sessions of repeating down the same ineffective track. You may recall that Monica (who had social anxiety but, beneath that, core beliefs of incompetence and fears of maturing) was avoiding certain topics in consultations, which needed to be discussed constructively. This could be achieved naturally by an alert therapist who is willing to say out aloud things they sense or observe in the therapy room. However, formal monitoring of therapy processes would enable an efficient and candid discussion of therapy.

Finally, in Neil's presentation with depression, his initial negative beliefs about the ability to change one's thinking style and mood could be discussed as early as possible. The day that Neil brings his wife into the session without warning or planning is also a high risk for alliance rupture — he may be resentful that she insists on coming or may fear the therapist judging him for not having been more truthful about his drinking. Any such emotion and any intrusion upon the working alliance needs to be discussed (and it is the therapist's responsibility to broach these conversations). A therapist might also have strong emotions about Neil's extramarital affair, especially if that therapist can identify with his wife or the younger woman at work. The ability to notice our own emotions and to manage our interactions with Neil at this time will be crucial to the ongoing alliance and therefore effectiveness. There will be time in the future to Socratically explore with Neil the choices that he made. But the initial response needs to be an impassive listening process without either judgement or forgiveness of those choices.

## Noticing and managing ruptures

In any therapy process there is likely to be a rupture in the fabric of the TA. This could manifest in many ways, such as subtle shift in affect in the client, telephoning later to cancel the next session, or a more obvious declaration from the client such as, 'you don't get it'. One of the reasons for such a gap in the alliance is that the client perceives the therapist hasn't been attuned to them the way they expect. Naturally, this could be a problem with their expectations — some clients have a sensitised need for validation from their developmental years (Leahy, 2006). But it could also be due to poor listening on the part of the therapist or actually their failure to communicate or demonstrate how well they have indeed been listening. The average therapy session requires much intellectual work. When the therapist is working hard to recall details about the client's history, develop an ICF, and suppress some ideas while developing others in their head, then these intellectual tasks can easily interfere with the core therapeutic task of making the client feel that we respect them, are attuned to them and care about them. A therapist is well advised to practice self-monitoring and self-regulation such that they can do the internal work while also externalising a demonstration of validating attunement of their client. When the therapist catches themselves pensive and perhaps not responding to the client, while they process ideas and hypotheses, it can be helpful to inform the client. An example might be, 'what you said made me think a lot — please let me make a note about that before we continue'.

Regardless of the cause, all therapists can have moments when our clients feel misunderstood or not 'heard'. It is the therapist's responsibility to be vigilant for these ruptures and then manage them. An effective therapist will be comfortable with pausing the session and enquiring about what the client might be feeling or thinking at that point in time. So much can be gained from such discussions. In doing so, that therapist can communicate to the client that this is a safe place to discuss feelings and that they can tolerate negative feedback from the client about the therapy process — indeed they welcome it. Thus, the therapist 'socialises' the client to the therapy process. We can't expect a client to know how to make therapy effective — that is the role and responsibility of the therapist. (See Chapter 7 for a summary on keeping CBT on track and effective, as well as client guidelines for therapy). It is also an opportunity to start to explore early maladaptive schemas, which will impact all relationships. How the client responds to the therapist and the difficult emotions that emerge in a session is a reliable indicator of their core beliefs and their response style with other people in their life.

In this regard, the core cognitive therapy skills of curious and collaborative enquiry (through strategic questioning) can be helpful. Questions that the therapist could use to respectfully and constructively draw attention to the reactivity and emotionality include: *'I noticed a change just then. Can I ask what you were thinking and feeling a few moments ago?'*.

If the client denies having any emotions then normalising and validating before pursuing a little further might be warranted:

> *I was wondering if you were feeling annoyed or surprised that I didn't acknowledge the big importance of what you just said. In hindsight, I guess I skipped on to another topic quickly. I think many people would feel at least surprised that we didn't discuss it further — maybe even hurt or disappointed. If you have any of those natural emotions, then I think it would be helpful to acknowledge them and we can take time to repair that. That is what we have to do in therapy to keep our work effective.*

> *Can I ask . . . have you had that feeling before? ... With whom? ... How often does it occur? ... Can you recall the very first time that feeling really hit you?*

> *What connections or conclusions can we draw from this that would be helpful for you in the future with other people?*

> *This might happen again in one of our sessions. Even though I work hard to listen well and I will always work to get the best results for you, I can be too eager to get on to certain topics, such that I might miss things. I hope you will be able to give me this sort of helpful feedback in the future.*

Just like the process of building the size and strength of a muscle is said to be one of 'tear and rebuild', through exertion and recovery, so the therapeutic bond can get deeper and stronger by the willingness of both parties to move to the discomfort and work through it, rather than avoid or skim over it.

### Helpful therapist cognitions

- *It pays to drop the agenda item in therapy to address emotionality or a breach in the therapeutic alliance; after all, without the alliance, there will be no therapy worth doing.*

- *It is my responsibility to manage the session, including client emotions.*

- *I seek out and welcome strong emotions in session. Having strong emotions in the room is an opportunity to:*

  *(a) learn more about my client, and*

  *(b) demonstrate that emotions can be tolerated and discussed then managed.*

- *A difficulty in the therapeutic relationship is:*

  *(a) to be expected at some stage, so I'll be alert to it*

  *(b) an opportunity to protect the therapy potency, and*

  *(c) an opportunity to help the client learn about how they react to other relationships in their life.*

- *It is helpful to acknowledge that I inadvertently contributed to them not feeling appreciated, connected with me or understood by me. We can explore what that feeling was like before rectifying it and moving on.*

- *Feedback from my client about the quality of our TA is probably going to be helpful and worth the time gathering that data.*

## Unhelpful therapist cognitions

- *I won't bring that up or challenge the client because it might make them feel uncomfortable or embarrassed (and we can't let that happen).*

- *I don't want to set a precedent of them criticising me; anyway, I feel more comfortable when we have an agenda that gets followed every session.*

- *If I analyse every emotional change that I see in the client, then I won't have time for the actual therapy.*

- *I'm out of my depth talking about the therapeutic relationship.*

- *This is CBT not transference-focused psychodynamics.*

## Resistance

Some level of resistance and ambivalence in therapy is the norm. The most common reasons for ambivalence about engaging in CBT include experiential and emotional avoidance and fear of how hard the treatment is (especially for anxiety disorders and any trauma content). If the rationale for certain treatments has not been made sufficiently clear this may also cause ambivalence. Beyond this common 'ambivalence' is 'resistance' — a concept that needs to be viewed through the lens of compassionate understanding of the client's emotional and cognitive status, rather than accusing them of deliberately resisting your help. After all, when a person is in pain, they will naturally do what they can to alleviate that pain. Consider both physical and emotional pain. There are many ways to reduce or manage pain and some options are healthier than others. The healthier ones often take longer to be effective and require more effort. Their awareness of, capacity for, or willingness to try, certain self-management manoeuvres may not be sufficient for the work that you want to do, which will manifest as 'resistance'. And if that person cannot do that work (because they do not know what to do or how to do it or because the unhealthy options are the only ones role-modelled to them), then this is not their fault. It is the therapist's task to help them move to a slightly higher level of readiness to engage in that healthier work.

Most therapists naturally find themselves having natural reactions to this (such as frustration or demoralisation), which has the potential to affect the therapeutic relationship and alliance. Therefore, as soon as a therapist can bring nonjudging curiosity to the observed impasse, the more effective they will become. Some key techniques to manage client ambivalence and role with resistance are expanded in Chapter 5.

## Case studies

Our example of **Neil**, with depression, can provide an illustration of client ambivalence and the tasks that the therapist must negotiate not to make any resistance stronger through their own responses. A female therapist noticed that she had some automatic thoughts and emotional responses to hearing of Neil's had had an extramarital affair with a junior at work and how, after a long period of stating he would leave his wife for her, decided against this. These emotions were quite obvious to her, so she was able to put them aside and convey a sense of acceptance of Neil. But it was hard work. This therapist chose a deliberate compassionate exercise that kept her working on Neil's side. She reflected — at first outside the session and then with Neil in a session — on what factors made it understandable that he took these actions. Initially, Neil said that being a 'bad person' accounted for all his decisions. The therapist was able to say that she did not agree and they could explore his feelings of guilt and work towards a fuller understanding. Our therapist wanted to utilise these emotions therapeutically and so posed these questions to him:

> *Neil, if you are so unforgiving on yourself, then what impact does this have on your mood and your ability to be the father and husband that you are striving to be everyday now?*

> *Could you give yourself permission to focus on doing well by your values in the future, rather than focusing on the past that you can no longer alter?*

> *Given that you can be so unforgiving about yourself, does that mean you fear judgement by others — you know, assuming that others will judge you the way you do? … In fact, have you ever worried about what I might think about you? If so, we should talk*

*about that. So far, have your fears been strengthened to any degree or perhaps proven false?*

*I think it shows wisdom and courage to bring these issues up in therapy; and also a commitment to the collaborative process of functioning better. Can you see why I would see it that way?*

Let us also examine some of the interactions between **Amanda** and her therapist. Amanda continues to worry that she might actually collapse or faint or hurt someone else when she has an anxiety attack. Amanda's therapist is thinking: *'You have never once done these things in all your anxiety episodes and I have repeated the psychoeducation about the nature and safety of anxiety too many times already. Why can you not accept that anxiety is just unpleasant and not dangerous?!?'.* The therapist notices frustration towards Amanda as the main emotion, then notices some doubting thoughts and worry that they have missed something or have not done the CBT well enough.

Having noticed these thoughts and feelings as counter-transference, the therapist wisely wonders (a) what is it like for Amanda and (b) does she relate to other people or act in other situations the same way? A helpful hypothesis about clinician emotions of frustration and powerlessness is that the client has a need for others to take responsibility or take care of them.

The therapist decides to ask Amanda where she feels she is up to in her therapy goal of no longer fearing anxiety attacks, so they can wonder about this together. The hypothesis that she needs others to take control is not confirmed by her responses. Rather, Amanda says that she wants to be more functioning and wants to get better on her own — but the main problem is that her mind keeps doubting things and worrying despite the overwhelming evidence. This enables the therapist to name and explore the hypothesis of 'intolerance of uncertainty'.

Amanda guesses accurately: *'You must be really frustrated with me; you don't have to keep seeing me if you don't want to'.* How would you respond to that is session? This therapist decides to be constructively partly honest: *'I am not frustrated with you at all. I am glad to have the opportunity to talk about feelings. The only feeling I have is that I empathise with **your** frustra-*

*tion because I see how hard you are working but you keep getting stuck because of the obsessional doubt and your mind wanting you to be sure. Let's spend the rest of the session and probably a lot of the next few appointments working on strategies to break through the fear you experience when your mind tells you that you need to be 100% sure that NOTHING bad can possibly happen'.*

## Working on your therapeutic relationships

How exactly do you convey warmth and a positive regard to your client?

Would you find the following statements acceptable for some or all of your clients?

*I was thinking quite a bit about you and your therapy since our last session and I wanted to raise one or two of the issues that we were working on again.*

*It's good to see you. I was looking forward to our appointment to see what it was like for you to tackle those homework ideas.'*

*I admire the way you are bringing real emotional honesty and a type of authenticity to this therapy process.*

*I think that you have far more positive qualities than you give yourself credit for. For instance, my perception of you is that you're thoughtful and kind, perceptive, hard working and creative in your own lovely ways. Can we discuss what makes it hard for you so say these things to yourself or even hear them from someone?*

What are the advantages and concerns about these various therapist statements? What might make you hold back from letting your client know that you think positively towards them?

The common reasons why therapists hold back from conveying warmth are understandable but can be managed through self-awareness, then willingness to challenge and test out predictions and assumptions. These might include:

- Concern about injecting one's own emotions and opinions into the therapy space.

- Being busy in the session holding competing hypotheses and considering which therapeutic strategy or task to address next and then how to do that optimally.

- A supervisor once told them not to.

- Concern that the client will get the wrong message or they will establish unwanted positive or even erotic transference towards the therapist.

All of these concerns can be managed such that the therapist can feel free to express positive regard for their client in appropriate ways for that client in that setting.

## Is there a risk of overemphasising the TA?

This chapter has invited CB therapists to evaluate the priority that they place on forming a powerful TA and their skilfulness to do so successfully. It is important, though, not to exalt or lionise the TA as being the main or only therapeutic ingredient. Beck et al. (1979) mention the TA as being necessary for therapeutic effectiveness. But the same authors say that it is not sufficient and place greater emphasis on therapeutic techniques and interventions to create efficient change. Indeed, the cardinal shift for Beck — a psychoanalytically trained psychiatrist — was to provide depressed clients with discrete, learnable techniques for changing their mood. While plenty of research, alluded to above, supports the role of the TA, some meta-analytic studies have shown weak correlations between strength of TA and therapy effectiveness (Martin, Garske, & Davis, 2000). An excessive belief in the TA as a therapeutic source of change may lead the therapist to use a low dose of cognitive therapy, thus weakening effectiveness (Waller & Turner, 2016). Similar ideas are explored further in Chapter 7 for staying on track in therapy.

# Highlights and take-home messages

1. Therapist variables contribute to outcomes and these variables are known and modifiable

2. Talk about and attend to the relationship explicitly in helpful ways, depending on the client

3. Find appropriate ways to convey warmth and a positive regard to each client

4. Work at every session to monitor and modify your own thoughts and feelings about the therapy process and the client to show nonjudging curiosity and empathy

5. Be willing to pause and discuss even minor ruptures in the working alliance

6. A weak therapeutic alliance often leads to poorer outcomes or premature termination, so it pays dividends to take therapy time to do this.

# Chapter 4

# Understanding and maintaining motivational dynamics

Act as if what you do makes a difference. It does.

William James

People often say that motivation doesn't last. Well, neither does bathing — that's why we recommend it daily.

Zig Ziglar

Our case study of Amanda, with panic disorder, can help to illustrate some of the common factors affecting motivation for better and for worse. She is initially engaged with CBT but, with time, becomes very reluctant to repeat the interoceptive exposure on her own at home and she very rarely follows the suggested homework tasks (such as driving her car a little more each week, according to the fear-hierarchy that she and her therapist established for her agoraphobic avoidance). She is at risk of dropping out.

To what degree is it the therapist's *role* or even *responsibility* to increase her motivation to do the work that will get her better? Should a client be free to decline one or more part of recommended treatment? The answer to that final question is a clear affirmative. The answer to the former, though, needs a thorough examination.

And what about Monica? She is the student with core assumptions about being incompetent and unlikeable and so is very scared to function in the world. Naturally, she exercises avoidance of many life events but also of topics in therapy that make her feel unsafe or uncomfortable. Her avoidance is so habitual that she barely notices it. Is it her right only to work on the topics that she chooses? After all, it is her therapy isn't it? To what degree do you think the therapist has a role — maybe a responsibility — to help Monica to address the emotions, thoughts and behaviours that she finds uncomfortable?

These examples illustrate the need to start thinking about whose responsibility is it to work on motivational balance in therapeutic work. There are no absolute right or wrong ways to consider this. It depends very much on the assessment of the causes of a client's ambivalence about treatment. For instance, if your questioning reveals that Amanda is reluctant to do more exposure interventions because of a fear of 'I would not cope; I might fall to pieces and never recover', then you would probably be inclined to address this fear in therapy, rather than accept this as her *choice* and not try to do effective treatment. Your position on responsibility for managing motivation might be affected by other workplace-specific factors; for instance, whether your service has long waiting lists, if you have a limited number of sessions possible within your service, or if you typically conduct therapy in group format.

It is well known that a client's motivation to work hard in therapy naturally goes up and down and is rarely at 100%, and is influenced by variables that can be discovered and altered in the counselling process. Within individual CBT, the responsibility for managing fluctuations in motivation needs to be shared by the client and the therapist, with the therapist taking the leading role, as they will understand the therapy and emotional variables better. Ultimately, though, it is up to the client because therapy is not imposed on the client — it is always respectful of their limits and wishes.

# What is motivation?

Motivation is defined as 'a driving force or forces responsible for the initiation, persistence, direction, and vigour of goal-directed behaviour' (Coleman, 2015). In therapeutic terms, a more helpful construct is 'willingness'. In our own lives, most of us have countless instances of plans, good intentions and self-made promises that never get enacted. Equally, we can all think of activities that we have undertaken that we found arduous, maybe even aversive, but we did them. Examples might include undergoing an invasive medical procedure, seeing your dentist, studying for an exam, or attending a certain social event. As you think of your examples, were you 'motivated' to do that activity? Did you *want* to do it? Chances are that you *wanted* a certain outcome and were therefore *willing* to endure or participate in the process.

Being respectful of and compassionate towards a client's motivational blockages and mixed feelings is important for many reasons. The therapist needs to role-model compassion, so the client can internalise self-compassion. It also helps the therapist to find the right pace, which protects the working alliance. Understanding a client's level of ambivalence about what seems objectively in their interest can be achieved by:

- listening actively to your clients and asking questions designed to reveal personal reasons for them to work hard, as well as understanding the factors that naturally erode their willingness to do the work

- recalling your own past experiences of when you have worked hard at an arduous task and when you decided to cease that goal

- reading clinical accounts of other clients.

### If my client has decided to come for treatment, why are they not more motivated?

People do the best they can with their own resources before they ask for help. A person's decision to come to treatment signifies that their distress levels exceeded their personal threshold for help-seeking. At some point, though, they may dip below that threshold again. This could happen between calling for an appointment and coming to their first consultation (in which case, they may not keep that appointment or will come with mixed feelings about the appointment). There are various other reasons they can get to a point below their threshold of bothering to get help when in the midst of therapy. Perhaps they start to feel better, or the therapy they have started may feel more like hard work, or take longer, or is more expensive than they predicted.

Motivation is dynamic and fluid, so we ought to expect it will change over time. If you are familiar with the variables that most commonly impact willingness to pursue treatment, you are more likely to hypothesise accurately about each client and discuss it openly with them.

### What are the main variables that influence motivation to work hard in therapy?

There are many factors that can influence a person's motivation or willingness to engage in each part of CBT. Some relate to psychopathology, including worthlessness (that could be associated with major depression or an early maladaptive schema of defectiveness) and hopelessness (as a symptom of depression). These factors can be addressed through psychoeducation, including this in the ICF and then actively treating those symptoms with cognitive therapy and behavioural activation.

Beyond depression there are very many other factors that can be reduced down to three major components: the importance or value that we place on a certain outcome or process; a personal cost–benefit analysis of change compared to the status quo; and self-efficacy, or the confidence that we can make a specific behavioural change. These factors are graphically represented in Figure 4.1, which could be used as a psychoeducational tool if motivation and willingness needed to be discussed explicitly.

Also refer to Appendix A for an example of a tool that can be used whenever a client is stuck or ambivalent. This tool consists of four lines — four visual analogue scales — on which the client rates four variables for one specific behaviour. The scales are: (1) the importance of doing that behaviour and this pertains to congruence with values; (2) the perceived benefits of doing this specific behaviour; (3) the perceived costs of doing the same behaviour; and (4) the client's confidence that they can do this behaviour.

For example, in Neil's case, the therapist and he have been discussing the reasons to start to set some simple limits with his daughter. The target action or behaviour for this exercise is for him to talk to his daughter in the

**Factors that influence our motivation for action**

Determination
Importance in my life

Perceived losses or
negatives of change

Perceived benefits to
me of change

Confidence that
I can do it

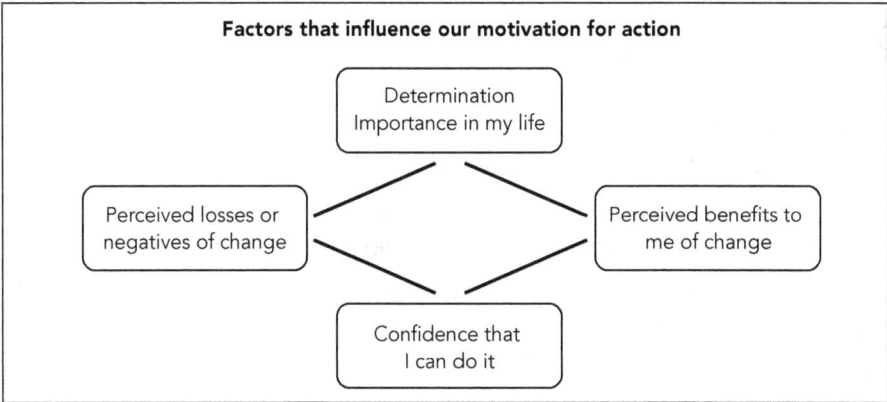

**FIGURE 4.1**
Factors that influence our motivation for action.

next fortnight and let her know that she will from now on have a fixed allowance and that she needs to manage her own budget within that generous allowance — he cannot and will not pay for anything more. Neil's rating on the first scale is 80% (which the therapist feels is high enough and so not much further discussion is had other than asking Neil to explain why it is so high — which helps to reinforce this strength). Neil rates the benefits as 60% and the costs at 75%. His confidence that he can have the conversation as planned is 50%. These ratings make it clear to Neil's therapist that the suggested behaviour is not an appropriate goal at this stage and so that therapist takes time to explore what those perceived costs are, hoping to see if there are some faulty predictions that could be disputed or tested somehow. Likewise, the confidence ratings are addressed at some length.

These four visual analogue scales (Appendix A) can be very useful and efficient whenever a client seems stuck or is 'resistant'. Therefore, let's look at another example — this time, Monica, with social anxiety, anxiety attacks and worry. The therapist thinks that it will be helpful if Monica attends some relatively easy social situations and practices her new coping strategies while she tests out the validity of her anxiogenic thoughts and predictions. The target behaviour is turning up to a seminar on campus and arriving 15 minutes early such that she may have the opportunity to start a conversation with someone she knows there. Monica rates the importance of this at 50%. She also rates the perceived cost at 66% and the possible benefits at 33%. Her self-efficacy or confidence rating that she can do this in the next fortnight is 40%. The most striking rating is the 50% importance — which most therapists would see as being low. It means that Monica perhaps does not see a connection with this therapy exercise and her own desired outcomes. Or, in Monica's case, she does not actually want to become functionally independent. This would become the main focus of therapeutic attention, with the therapist asking more about what she does want for herself and what changes might move her in that direction. With this data at hand, the therapist might be quicker to get to the hypothesis of maturity fears. Her low ratings on benefits and confidence could also be explored.

As a general guide, all positive ratings need to be 70% or above (and the costs perceived as less than 50%) before the therapist and client agree to trial the target behaviour.

## Understanding readiness to change

A very helpful model of a person's motivation or readiness to change their behaviour is the Stages of Change model or Transtheoretical Model of readiness for change first developed by Prochaska and DiClemente (1983). The essence of their model is that not all people who consult a health professional are ready to take active steps to change a specific behaviour. Prochaska and DiClemente developed their model to help understand the way different smokers think and feel about quitting but it can apply quite well to any behaviour. They found that most people can be said to be in one of four stages of readiness for change before moving into maintenance or perhaps relapse: precontemplation, contemplation, preparation and action

For the CB therapist, this heuristic model has both limitations and powerful benefits. The key implications are discussed below.

### 1. Do not assume your client is in an Action stage of readiness for change for all behaviours and all aspects of treatment

For example, Amanda has panic disorder. She is willing to do some interoceptive exposure with you in session but her fear levels remain very high and her danger expectancies do not alter over time. She is very reluctant to repeat the interoceptive exposure on her own at home and she very rarely follows the homework tasks. Thus, we could say that she is in an 'Action stage of readiness for change' for doing some treatment activities but in a 'Contemplative stage' for other therapeutic actions. The therapist would not keep pushing for *all* behavioural goals or experiments. Rather, the therapist would shift the attention to learning collaboratively about why it makes sense for Amanda that she is reluctant to do more and gauging how near or far she is to action-oriented interventions. It should then be possible to find an appropriate therapeutic task for her at this point in time. That task would help her to move towards greater readiness for the most potent (and, for her, the scariest) CBT interventions.

### 2. Align your interventions with the client's stage of readiness for change for each presenting issue or behaviour

If Amanda does not want to take the risk of not coping with anxiety, then the intervention needs to slow down and could instead target her fear of anxiety at a tolerable pace. It might be very helpful if the therapist were to describe a temporary therapy approach that relies more on cognitive restructuring than behavioural exposure, and equally helpful to let her know that they believe that a careful collaborative process will definitely help her. Suggesting a smaller behavioural goal and helping Amanda experience some success or mastery might be the most motivating thing. However, a good CB therapist will also be sensitive to her capacity to cope and her willingness to engage in therapeutic steps so small that they seem inconsequential. Many therapists would also successfully suspend the focus on treating panic per se and devote session-time to the broader issue of Amanda's intolerance of negative emotions — often referred to as 'experiential avoidance'. Table 4.1 summarises the therapist's tasks for each major stage of readiness for change.

### 3. A poor alignment of stage of readiness for change and intervention chosen by the therapist can increase resistance and harm the TA

Pushing ahead with standard CBT (which is an action-oriented treatment), may make the client feel that you are disregarding their feelings and what they are saying to you (verbally or nonverbally). If this is the case, then, at best, the CBT intervention will not be effective. At worst, you can create a distancing — a gap in the therapeutic relationship. Imagine if you kept asking Amanda to find a way to do the same home-based tasks. It is not likely that she will do it, creating a potential for her to feel hopeless about

## TABLE 4.1
Therapist's tasks for each stage of readiness for change

| Signs that a person is in this stage | The therapist's task(s) in this stage |
| --- | --- |

### Precontemplation

| | |
| --- | --- |
| • Denying the seriousness or impact of the status quo | Work on developing your alliance and engagement. |
| • Changing the topic | Give voice to their sentiment about change and not changing in a validating, accepting way. |
| • Avoiding treatment | Normalise and validate their reasons to stay as they are; validate their fears and concerns about change. |
| • Declining suggestions for help | |
| • Defensiveness | Seek permission to learn more about them and their reasons for feeling the way they feel. |
| | Ask if they are '100% content' with how things are. |
| | Identify their values (especially those that help to understand why they do not change, as well as those that might give them reason to change) |
| | Socratic questions designed to help them see the gap between habitual choices and where their values would take their life. |

### Contemplation

| | |
| --- | --- |
| • Inconsistent homework or attendance | Validate their stance and the fact that they have mixed feelings and desires (ambivalence). |
| • Expressing fluctuating or mixed feelings about their condition and treatment | Normalise this.

Empathise with why that person is thinking about change but not yet feeling safe or ready to change. |
| • Statements like 'maybe, I'm not sure' or 'yeah — I know I should, but ...' | Discuss what could be done about the perceived dangers of change. |
| | Amplify negatives of the status quo through Socratic questions. Similarly, highlight potential benefits of changing. Juxtapose different aspects of their ambivalence (e.g., top 2 reasons to change and top 2 reasons not to). |
| | Find out what they ARE willing to work on ... generate progressively smaller tasks or goals until their confidence reaches a threshold for action. |
| | Contract to work on healthy ways to meet their needs, even if they continue to also resort to a problematic way to meet their needs. |
| | Ask if they'd be willing to do an experiment to test out one or more assumptions (e.g., the prediction that they would not cope without carrying diazepam with them; or speaking up once at work). |

**Table 4.1** continued

---

### *Preparation*

| | |
|---|---|
| • They have decided that they wish to change but have not quite yet started | Continue to normalise and validate ambivalence. Work together to lower any concerns about change that they still have. |
| • A high desire for a new outcome but lacking the knowledge or confidence to achieve that outcome | Inform and educate about treatment options. |

Increase self-efficacy through:

- others' experiences
- own past experiences
- using a consistent therapy model together.

Safe experimentation when ready; start with small achievable steps; hypothesis testing.

Anticipate drops in motivation and discuss how they can remain *willing* when things get tough.

---

### *Action*

| | |
|---|---|
| • The client is taking steps to engage in treatment or change a specific behaviour | Do the cognitive and behavioural interventions that come from your assessment and formulation — but be mindful that motivation can drop. Anticipate challenges and ask the client to generate a list of future outcomes and values-based ideas that will help keep them on track. |

---

### *Maintenance*

| | |
|---|---|
| • They have achieved one or more goal and do not feel the need to change that further | Increase the likelihood of retaining this change by: |

- asking questions to highlight how good it feels to have this outcome

- asking what it would feel like if they regressed in the future

- investing in a relapse-prevention plan based on their history of symptoms. A good relapse prevention plan is informed by the client's ICF and by establishing the likely high-risk situations, knowing their early warning signs and having contingencies rehearsed.

These contingencies can include looking at a list of the values-based reasons for maintaining their gains, safety manoeuvres (like where to go or who to be with) and helpful beliefs to re-assert.

---

recovering and wondering what is wrong with her — but not getting the help to address that.

### 4. Your task is to shift the client one step closer towards 'Action'

This can sometimes be done with cognitive or behavioural techniques and sometimes motivational techniques. In Amanda's case, the therapist takes time to ask with curiosity all the reasons why she does not feel like repeating the interoceptive exposure on her own. They empathise with her fear of 'not coping' and 'losing control and never recovering' with a statement like: *'That is a terrifying thought — of going crazy forever if you can't cope. That helps me understand'*. Then the therapy shifts to addressing her fears: *'I want you to know, though, that I think that together we can overcome those understandable fears. Why don't we keep talking about that today? I'm going to ask you to work out with me what you mean by 'not coping' and what your fears are'*.

For Amanda, many of her fears might be reduced by a combination of (a) psychoeducation about 'coping well enough' and how anxiety is a safe and adaptive response to perceived threat and (b) reflecting on existing evidence that she has never lost control or gone crazy no matter how anxious she ever became. Then the therapist can ask her if she would be willing to help devise some new tests to disprove her residual fears about what might happen if she got anxious when on her own. The motivational work can be woven into the fabric of the cognitive therapy with questions such as: *'Remind me what brought you to therapy — how does the anxiety disorder interfere with life in the way you want to lead it?'* and *'what are the two greatest benefits that you will experience in your life once you have disproven your fears and they no longer feel believable?'*. Alternatively: *'This can feel scary and we all like to avoid feeling scared — but what are your reasons for going through these experiments?'*.

## Common reasons for ambivalence

There are as many reasons for ambivalence about change as there are clients, but there are some also recurring themes. The more we understand the common sources of ambivalence, the quicker we will be able to identify and empathise with our next client's experience. Here are some of the more common factors accounting for ambivalence about treatment.

- **The client is not aware that they can be helped.** For instance, many clients are not aware how common certain psychological conditions are, and what psychological treatments are available. Indeed, they may have been given misinformation by a doctor or a relative.

- **There is a misperception of therapy processes.** For example, a client may hold the belief, 'talking things out should be enough on its own'; or 'psychologists make their clients touch toilets to overcome OCD'.

- **Bad experiences with past therapy.** Examples may include engaging in therapy where there were poor boundaries and they felt confused about the process; or a client was required to enter a feared situation for planned systematic desensitisation when they were not willing or ready and had a panic attack, leaving them sensitised and with lower confidence.

- **Fear of distress.** For instance, a client has felt flooded before and pictures themselves crying uncontrollably during and after a therapy session; or perhaps they have always been averse to emotional discomfort and have an array of habitual methods to 'medicate' negative affect.

- **Metacognitions that make a person reluctant to change.** In the case of PTSD a person may think 'if I reassure myself that the chance of being assaulted again is actually fairly low, that will mean I take risks and it could EASILY happen again'. A person with an eating disorder thinks 'I need to tell myself how greedy and disgusting it is to have a full lunch, otherwise I'll lose my ability to control my weight'. Someone with panic disorder, like Amanda, might think 'my sense of danger must mean something important — so I need to attend to my feelings and be guided by them'.

- **Secondary gain or functional outcomes.** For example, a client feels safe now that others have assumed their domestic responsibilities; or another gets a sense of unique identity and inner strength from their ability to stay at work until 10 pm, but this makes them isolated and depressed. In the case of Monica, she discovered that suffering anxiety and appearing to struggle with her mood meant that a parent took greater care of her, which she found reassuring and safe.

- **Fusion with an early maladaptive schema.** In Monica's case, she truly believes (as a fact) that she is less competent than others. To act in a way that opposes this feels wrong, undeserving and frightening. Another client feels that they are so worthless that they do not deserve to feel better and they are not allowed to work on activities that could lead to feeling better.

Each of these issues can be addressed via building a case formulation, psychoeducation, some motivational enhancement or working out which cognitive or behavioural interventions might be helpful — depending on the circumstances and the client details.

## Key strategies to build motivation

The following strategies comprise a summary of the literature from motivational interviewing (Miller & Rollnick, 2009; 2012; Moyers & Rollnick, 2002; Westra, Aviram, & Doell, 2011; Westra & Dozois, 2006), acceptance and commitment therapy (ACT; Hayes, Strosahl & Wilson, 2011), self-determination theory (Vansteenkiste, Williams, & Resnicow, 2012) and behavioural therapy principles (Waller, 2012).

Before techniques and procedures are examined, it is worthwhile highlighting that the *tone* of these approaches is arguably more important than the *content* of the interaction. We need to strike a tone that is nonjudging and curious, so the client feels validated and eager to collaborate in a process of enquiry into why they find making certain changes hard. The therapist does not lecture and tell them in which ways they would be 'better off'. Rather, even if it takes three times as long, a series of open questions can be used to elicit from the client *their* reasons to keep the status quo and *their* reasons for change. The therapist guides this process with deliberate intent to tip the balance of motivation and then, when they feel the client is ready, ask for a commitment to work on one piece of behaviour that is consistent with their valued outcomes that the client believes they can do. Respect for the client's autonomy and intelligent personal choices pervades the process and yet the same therapist can ask how their thinking makes sense if it appears not to. If the TA is strong enough, the therapist can ask probing questions without it feeling like judgement.

## 1. Help your client to achieve early behavioural changes

Achieving some change early in therapy is one of the more important ways to enhance the TA and build a client's willingness to work collaboratively. As mentioned above, motivation for the hard work of therapy goes up and down and is rarely around 100%. That does not mean a therapist necessarily needs to invest a lot of time doing motivational enhancement work. Even when some ambivalence is present, it may be possible to find a therapeutic task that the client can do. This task needs to meet just two main criteria: (a) it seems personally relevant — that is, it is consistent with their desired outcomes that they stated in the assessment process, and (b) their self-efficacy for doing the task is high enough, which means that a range of options needs to be discussed until the client feels 'confident enough' to engage in the task.

A CB therapist will be accustomed to using a 'fear hierarchy' – that is, a scale or hierarchy of perceived difficulty and altering variables to reach a point where the client definitely can participate in the process. It is important to capitalise on any small changes and efforts with some reflection on what was achieved. The post-task discussion is designed to elicit and amplify feelings of achievement, mastery and of optimism about further gains. At the same time, the client should be sensing that their therapist is attuned to them, the proposed therapy seems to be effective, and they have the capacity to do what it takes to get better. Thus, their willingness to work hard can increase while the TA is strengthened.

Waller (2012) has highlighted some important caveats about doing motivational interventions and, while his article pertains to eating disorders, it has some applicability to other conditions. He suggests that verbal statements of motivational status and readiness for change are unreliable compared to actual behaviours. He also cites research that changes occurring early in therapy (a) predict long-term improvement and (b) increase both motivation and the perceived bond with the therapist. He recommends that motivational interventions that include values-based discussions be woven throughout therapy and that it helps to set firm boundaries and expectations for change early.

## 2. Shift the focus to motivational status

Signs of ambivalence within treatment are numerous and could include behaviours such as frequent cancelling or deferring of appointments, incomplete homework activities, reluctance to talk about certain topics, or hesitation with some therapy activities. If your client's ambivalence is strong and it is not easy to make any early gains, then it is helpful to find a way to discuss this constructively. One of the key mottos in therapy is 'say out aloud what is happening but yet to be articulated'. Yet we do not always articulate the observations about motivational balance for some understandable reasons. The therapist may have their own unhelpful assumptions or fears that can be disputed if tested out, such as 'my client will be offended if I say they don't seem to be motivated', or 'I need to get on with the actual treatment — that's my job'. There are ways to bring up motivational status in a nonjudging constructive way. Furthermore, if ambivalence goes unacknowledged and the therapist keeps finding ways to plough on, the client might feel invalidated and resistance may build. If the client agrees that they are not sure of their readiness to progress with this aspect of therapy, then one good option is to suggest spending some of the session-time discussing that directly, rather than continuing with the planned therapy agenda.

A therapist could state:

> *I sense some hesitation with this activity and I am sure that there is an understandable reason for that. Can I ask what mixed feelings you have about doing this activity?*

> *Most people get nervous or have some doubts before doing an exposure-based treatment session like we have planned. How are you feeling about it?*

> *You mentioned at our initial assessment that you wanted to talk about anger and verbal aggression because this was affecting your home relationships. But I have noticed that more recently you have said that this is no longer an issue. I also recall how uncomfortable it made you feel at the time — can I check whether you think it would be worth us bringing it up again at some stage even if it feels bad for a few minutes?*

Some clients come to an appointment with little or no readiness to change at all, such as those people required to attend by an employer, partner or parent. In these cases, it makes sense to talk explicitly about their motivational status from the start of the assessment process. For example, given all that has been stated thus far in this chapter, it would make sense to say:

> *So, I gather you are here at your mother's suggestion. I'd like to hear your thoughts and feelings about that.*

> *Given that your employer has required you to be here, we'd better start by discussing how much you **want** to be here and how much trust you have in talking to me.*

### 3. Empathise with each person's reasons for their ambivalence and hesitation

Clinicians commonly make an effort to understand a client's emotional state and share that understanding with them. When a client is 'stuck' in treatment or ambivalent about change, the focus of that understanding switches from *how they feel* to *why they are stuck*.

It can be very helpful at this stage to use statements that normalise ambivalence and validate their own mixed feelings. The therapist might use phrases such as:

> *You know, just about all my clients working on their self-worth find it hard to generate positive self-evaluations — it can feel like you are breaking an important rule that has worked for you.*

Equally:

> *I think I can understand why you are not sure about doing our planned behavioural experiment today — just about everyone doing this work finds that their mind starts predicting that it could go wrong or feel unbearably scary.*

Some other examples relating to our three clients follow shortly.

### 4. Build self-efficacy

Low confidence may be one of or even the main contributing factor to a person struggling with an aspect of treatment. Since the earliest contributions of Bandura (1977), it has been well understood that engagement in a behaviour is predicted by confidence that the person can do that behaviour and this confidence can be increased through established methods and steps.

It helps to assess self-efficacy directly. Many people use a visual analogue scale or a confidence rating as a percentage. When doing so, one needs to be behaviourally specific. Here are some examples using our case studies:

- **Neil** feels unable to decline any requests that his adult daughter makes for money. As an example of assessing self-efficacy, ask him:

  *On a scale from 0 to 100, how confident are you, that you could sit with your daughter and let her know that from now on, she will have a budget of $150 per week and it is up to her to learn to manage all her costs and needs within that budget?*

  *And would your confidence go up or down if you wrote out what you wanted to say as a letter first and then had that conversation? Would your confidence rating go up or down if your wife was present at the meeting?*

  *When we look at the rating you gave out of 100, what stops it from being 10 or 20 percentage points higher? For instance, are there specific fears that you have about that conversation not going well, or do you have worries about how she will react?*

- In another of our client cases, **Monica** agrees that it is time to test out her fears of being yelled at or judged negatively if she asked a lot of questions in a retail situation. Before heading to the shops together, you could ask:

  *How confident are you — on a scale from 0 to 100 — that you will be able to stay in the store and ask five questions of the retail assistant?*

And:

  *Our plan is for me to be next to you. What would be your confidence rating if I was standing by the entrance to the store and not by your side?*

Some established ways to increase a person's confidence that they can do certain behaviours include:

(a) **Behavioural approach strategies.** As noted above, making an early behavioural change is one of the most helpful ways to immediately increase a client's self-efficacy. Breaking down a behaviour or task into smaller steps or subgoals is very helpful. If you are using a fear hierarchy, suggest progressively smaller steps until the client has a self-efficacy rating of a specific behaviour of at least 70%.

(b) **Rehearsal.** Rehearsal is an extension of the behavioural approach strategies. A client can be encouraged to visualise themselves in the planned situation, using healthy coping strategies. It may also be possible initially to rehearse a healthy coping response in a much easier scenario.

(c) **Role modelling.** This technique is often done in CBT by the therapist doing the feared behaviour that the client fears as a prelude to the client's own effort. Alternatively, a client can be set a homework task to observe as many people as possible doing the target behaviour and making notes of what happens. Our client, Monica, could observe the therapist in a retail situation asking a series of questions and deliberately going slowly (designed to elicit worry that retail staff will be annoyed), or she could walk around a variety of shops and observe what happens when other people ask questions or leave tried-on clothes unfolded at the cashier and the like.

(d) **The-other-person test.** Invite the client to imagine that a close friend was about to embark on the same target behaviour. Then you can explore their confidence with questions such as, '*What advice would they give that other person?*', and '*So what is the difference between you and them?*'.

(e) **Reflecting on past efforts.** Ask the client if they can ever think of a time that they accomplished an action or task that they initially feared. Invite them to reflect on how this might apply here. If the client has had aversive learning experiences in the past, then these need to be acknowledged and addressed. One option would be to discuss the relevance of that past experience, as they may be making an 'over generalising thinking error'. The therapist can help the client weigh-up the pros and cons of testing this out again.

(f) **Address fears.** If you have used a few of the ideas presented above, then it should be possible through this process to identify the fearful predictions that lead to low confidence:

- In Neil's case, he shares a fear that his daughter will cry and she will become angry and withdraw. When asked to define 'withdraw', he says that he visualises her saying 'fine — then I'll never ask for anything from you' and walking away then not talking to him for days at a time. Any fears of a client can be addressed through the normal cognitive disputation and behavioural experimentation approaches that a CB therapist would be familiar with.

- Monica fears that if she keeps getting better, then her parents will no longer be as attentive, which means that she will not get the support that she needs. The therapist may draw on several possible approaches, including questioning the likelihood that her parents will react in the predicted way or even asking the parents to join a session to discuss these fears. Ultimately, though, Monica needs to start believing that she is actually more competent and capable than her core fears tell her, and that is likely to take several devoted consultations.

## 5. Identify the key values held by your client

This aspect of an intervention starts from the commencement of the initial assessment. *Values* are central to knowing your client. When any client gets stuck, it may be on account of one of their values. At the same time, though, it may be another value that provides them with the willingness to do hard work and tolerate high discomfort. It is therefore a beneficial investment in the therapy process to help the client understand the values in their life that influence their decisions and their motivational drives.

A value can be said to be some aspect of a person's self or life that they consider to be important. Honouring a life value typically leads to enhanced satisfaction and contentment and the inverse is true — when we contravene our values it is hard to feel content and we often feel pain.

There are several well-established methods to assess values and it is highly recommended that a clinician become familiar with options that are suited to the clinical populations that they work with most frequently.

Some accessible ways to identify values:

(a) **Selective listening to any themes that sound like life values.** On the understanding that values are central to behavioural and emotional change, we can start to look out for indirect statements such as: 'I want to spend more time …'; 'I feel so stupid when I …'; 'I go here most Sundays and every Thursday night'. For instance, if a client says they deeply regret not travelling as much or dropping out of their acting school, you might guess that they *value* travel and creativity in their life more than they *enact* it in their life.

(b) **Selective questioning when you hear 'change talk'.** If Neil were to say 'I keep promising myself that I will be firmer with my daughter', the therapist diverts the focus to that theme for some time with questions such as, *'Why do you say that?'; 'Why is that important to you?'; 'How good would it feel if you did make that change one day?'* or the like.

(c) **Listen out for, and enquire about, the best of times and the worst times.** These may be identified especially if the client has already mentioned a time when they felt either particularly joyful or in emotional pain. Start to explore what made them feel that way. Seek out a connection to a value — either the honouring or the contradiction of a value — and draw attention to that value.

(d) **Checklists.** Several are available online and in print form, mostly from the ACT literature (Hays et al., 2011). While Miller and Rollnick (2012) highlight the importance of identifying values, they offer less instruction on how to do this, compared with the creative and helpful ways offered in ACT texts. Many of the checklists are structured around major life domains, such as family, personal relationships, health, financial security, personal development and the like. In his book, *The Happiness Trap*, and the companion website, Harris (2007) provides some useful worksheets and a 'bull's eye' exercise to help clients consider how near or far certain behaviours are to one of their values.

(e) **Card-sort procedure.** It is possible to download or create your own list of value statements (e.g. adventurous; safe; generous; frugal; connected; career success; honour my family; honour my culture; look after my body; look after others; etc.). Clients are asked to sort these into two halves of lower and higher priority, according to what is the most important to them. Then they could be asked to select the top 50% of the top half already selected; or select their 'top 5' and rank these in priority. While you can use standardised cards, it is usually helpful to be able to write new ones for personal applicability.

(f) **The eulogy exercise (or birthday party exercise).** This is a well-established exercise designed to get the client to think about a time in the future and to reflect on what they want their whole life to have stood for. They are asked to imagine what the person delivering the eulogy (or speech) would say. Important variations include (a) if you were to die now, what would they say about how you *have* lived your life and (b) if you died well into the future what would you *like* them to say. The eulogy is very powerful because it reminds us that we have limited time and we get one go at living our life. However, this technique is ill-advised if the client is very depressed, has suicidal thoughts or is still a teen or child. That is when you can use a milestone birthday party instead.

(g) **Write about three people you admire and like.** In this exercise, a page is divided into three columns. At the top of each column, the client writes the names of three people they admire and respect, two of whom should be known to them. Under each name, they are asked to write in single words or short phrases what qualities this person possesses that makes them so admirable. This gives some insights into what the client values in a person and therefore themselves.

## 6. Develop a discrepancy between the client's current behaviour and the life that they value

If a client remains hesitant or very ambivalent about treatment, then it is possible to proceed with a series of Socratic questions to create some cognitive and emotional dissonance that may enhance their motivation for change. The dissonance is achieved by inviting the client to reflect on the congruence of a certain choice or behaviour, with specific goals (outcomes that they want) or with values (the person they want to be or the life they wish to lead). For this reason, it is crucial to have invested some time getting to know your client's values. As noted above, ACT resources (such as Harris, 2007) include some elegant worksheets to help a client examine the degree to which they are honouring their key values in certain life domains.

It can be more helpful, though, to be more behaviourally specific and tailor the exercise to each client, rather than use a generic worksheet. In Amanda's case, her valued outcomes include living independently, having a career and having a successful romantic relationship. Some of Neil's prominent values were to be the best father he could be, to maintain his physical health and to honour his sense of filial duty towards his aging parents. In each case the therapist could ask the client to rate the degree that some behaviours may serve or hinder one particular value on a scale (negative five [–5] to positive five [+5]). The completed values and ratings from Amanda are shown in Table 4.2. The completed values and ratings from Neil are shown in Table 4.3.

This exercise is a variation on the bull's eye exercise as cited in several ACT texts including Harris (2007). The bull's eye exercise involves asking a client how close or far any behaviour is to a nominated value, which is represented as an image of a target with concentric circles. The closer each behaviour is aligned to the value in question, the closer it is drawn to the bull's eye at the centre. Working through and discussing this exercise can also add to empathy and strengthen the TA. For an example, in Neil's case, the therapist has the opportunity to validate his efforts to be a good provider by devoting himself to his job. At the same time, they can express an understanding of the conflict of values — trying to be good at his job takes him away from his family.

## 7. 'Future Projection':

People are more willing to undertake actions that they find negative if they consider the future — either how *bad* things might be if they do not undertake that action, or how *good* the outcome might be if they do undertake that action.

Alongside your work identifying values, ask your client to conceive of a point in their future. The timeframe of that 'future projection' could be

## TABLE 4.2
Completed values and ratings of behaviours for Amanda.

**Value:** Being in an intimate romantic relationship

**Necessary Goals:** (a) being able to go on a date; (b) meeting existing friends at a bar; (c) learning not to fear anxiety.

| | |
|---|---|
| Catching a train with my sister | +4 |
| Catching a train on my own | +5 |
| Carrying Valium with me | −4 |
| Going to the supermarket on my own | +4 |
| Asking mum to drive me places | +4 −4 * |
| Choosing the quietest time of the day to go out | −1 |
| Only going to the shops when others can go with me | −3 |
| Going to coffee with friends | +5 |

* Amanda thought that getting mum to take her out was a positive step, as it enabled her to go out to places that she feared. On further reflection, she was able to see that it was such an avoidance of fear that it was holding her back as well as enabling her to go out a bit. Therefore, it was rated both helpful and unhelpful.

## TABLE 4.3
Completed values and ratings of behaviours for Neil.

**Value:** Being a good father

**Necessary Goals:** (a) coming home from work in time for dinner three times a week; (b) being less angry in my tone.

| | |
|---|---|
| Providing my children with a good lifestyle and comforts in life | +4 |
| Letting my daughter have whatever she what she wants | +5 |
| Letting both my children understand the value of money and teaching them how to budget | +5 |
| Having two alcohol-free days a week | −3 +3 * |
| Getting up early on Saturday to help with family activities | +4 |
| Staying at work until I feel that I have got everything done | −4 +2^ |
| Getting an alcoholic drink within 5 minutes of arriving home | −3 |
| Exercising more | +4 |
| Planning a 'date night' with my wife | +3 |

There are two double ratings from Neil.

* Neil said that if he did not drink, he would be more irritable; 'a few drinks help me to be a gentle relaxed guy'; but at the same time, he realised that it was not good role-modelling and that it made him more impulsive if he drank too much.

^ Neil also felt conflicted about leaving work, saying that one of his roles as father was to provide financial security for his family, which required him to stay at work; at the same time, being absent felt like a painful violation of the value of being 'a good dad'.

hours, days, or years. This timeframe depends on what the therapist believes is motivationally relevant and it is possible to ask the client what timeframe will work best for them. In order to elicit the client's reasons to change their behaviour, using our clients as examples, the therapist could perhaps ask:

> *With regard to this behaviour, if nothing were to change in the next six months, how would that feel?*

> *If you were able to make that change in the next few weeks, what would be the worst consequences for you? ... And what would be the best two or three consequences for you? How important would that be for you?*

> *If we got to the point where you no longer feared anxiety attacks, how would your life change?*

> *Amanda, we have discussed doing a specific monitoring task for the next seven days until our next appointment; what issues might interfere with you doing that? And what benefits might you get if you find a way to do it every day?*

> *Neil, inevitably, your daughter will turn 21, then 25 and then she will be in her 30s. What do you wish for her future attitude towards money and self-reliance?*

> *Monica, can you keep up the reliance on mum and dad for another year? What about three years? What about 15 years? What issues come up for you when I ask such questions?*

## 8. Roll with resistance

This is one of the key recommendations from Miller and Rollnick (2012) in their advice on doing motivational interviewing and their key idea is to avoid getting locked into debates, disagreements or arguments. It is possible to do this through a tone of respect for the client and being a willing listener to both 'change talk' (any mention of the desire to change or hope about change) and 'resistance talk' (any mention of reasons not to change, hopelessness or reasons to stay the same). Then, by using authentically curious questions, it is possible to learn more about the client. For instance, if Monica says, 'If I just stayed at home, then I wouldn't have any problems nor any anxiety', it may be tempting for the therapist to jump in with reasons to change or pointing out that staying at home actually is a problem in itself. Miller and Rollnick suggest a more elegant way of rolling with her momentum, like a master at one of the martial arts, by reflecting, *'Yep — your anxiety would be lower, which is what you want; but tell me about why you do choose not to stay at home all the time'*. Some additional ideas to roll with resistance include:

- **Offer a 'partial agreement'.** This is featured in Monica's example above. The task is to find something to agree with before shifting the conversation on to something more helpful or inviting a reflection. If Neil says that there is nothing wrong with drinking three to seven alcoholic drinks each evening and he seems to be fine drinking like this, the therapist could respond in several dozen ways; one might be: *'You've got a point — you do seem to be doing just fine. Do you mind, though if I ask a few more questions about your drinking, as there may be a chance that it is a maintaining factor for your depression, which is the main reason for you to seek help'*.

- **'Agree with a twist'.** This is a similar variant. In this case, the therapist responding to Neil might say, *'As you said, you seem to be functioning fine [pause] and does that mean you would function even better if you drank at the level recommended by your doctor?'*.

- **Deliberate exaggeration and 'the Devil's Advocate'.** If a client makes a statement that is congruent with not changing, another option is to exaggerate their position, with a view to them giving voice to the other side. With Monica the therapist might dare to say, *'In some ways that would be the perfect life — staying at home means that you would have no anxiety or hassles'*. In Neil's case the therapist might try *'Does that mean that there are no reasons at all to consider reducing your alcohol intake?'*. It is important to maintain a tone of authentic listening and empathising with their point of view in order to avoid sounding sarcastic or challenging.

- **Bring the client back to one of their stated goals.** A simple example might be simply, *'How do you think this relates to your main therapy goal, which is to reduce panic attacks?'*.

- **Explicitly redirecting the topic can also be done.** An example might be, '*I am not sure that continuing to discuss this in this way is the best use of your therapy session. By the end of this session, we both want you to feel that we have worked on the issues most important to you. What do you think we ought to spend our time on right now?*'.

## 9. Elicit a commitment to one or more new goals

It is crucial to seek a commitment from your client as soon as possible. The process of motivational enhancement can and ought to lead to the client electing to work on some therapy task or goal. This would hopefully be achieved within the session but for a client who is very stuck, it may take a more gradual process of working on other issues while time is taken to address the ambivalence for the more resistant issue. In Monica's case, she may be unwilling to tackle specific behavioural changes for some time but is willing to work on some schema-focused cognitive therapy to address her ideas that the world is hostile and she is neither equipped nor sufficiently competent as a young adult to survive.

## 10. Add it to your formulation

It is not only possible, but highly advantageous, to incorporate motivational dynamics into an ICF. This simultaneously adds additional layers of empathy, client insight, and inoculation against future resistance. The main ways that one seeks to add motivational factors to an ICF is to acknowledge (a) the costs and benefits of thinking or acting certain way, (b) the client's life values that may account either for their willingness to change or their inertia. Our case studies can illustrate this.

Let us remind ourselves how an early (end of initial assessment) case formulation looked for Amanda (See Figure 4.2). In version B, the motivational aspects are shown as large dotted lines (elements keeping her stuck) and small dotted lines (factors that may promote willingness to experiment with change even though she finds it scary).

Neil's ICF also serves as a useful example of adding some motivational data into an ICF and using that ICF to shift the motivational balance. This particular formulation is focused on his sense of being trapped into giving his younger daughter money and other resources beyond what he can

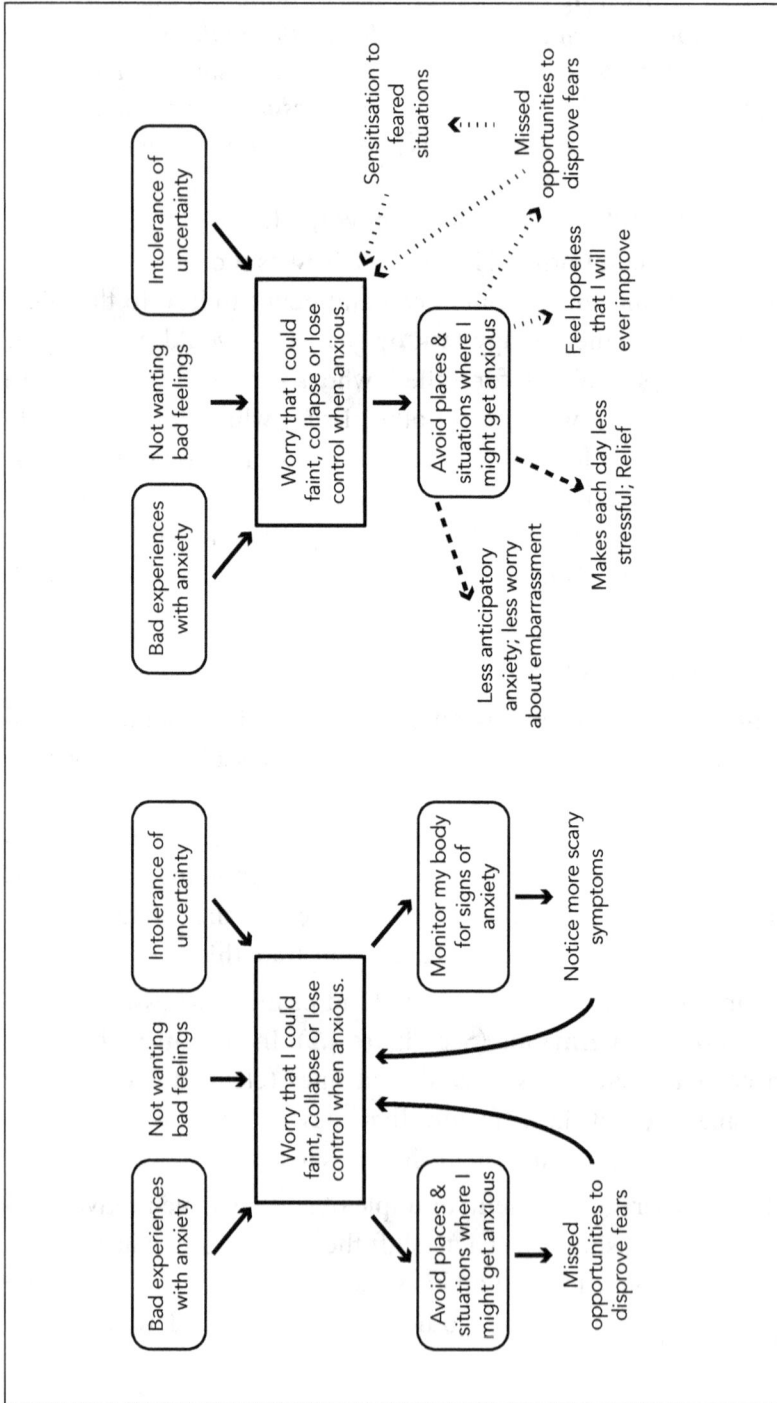

**FIGURE 4.2**
Version A (initial formulation for Amanda), and Version B (with motivational dynamic added).

really afford in the long-term and beyond what his other daughter receives. In Figure 4.3 you will see that some life values are added. These values are not connected causally with any arrow but are relevant. The therapist accepts and validates that Neil, as father, values being a good provider and a nurturer. The emotional focus is on his apprehensions about how his daughter will cope with any unhappiness on top of her significant mental health issues. The behavioural focus is on his lack of limits and never declining her requests, regardless of the cost to his mood or other relationships. Through the prism of his values and his past experiences, this is understandable. The therapist can enhance one of the steps advocated above — empathise with why the client is stuck. The therapist can add to this how the constant giving to his daughter feels more than 'good' — it feels 'right'. The associated reduction in anxiety is also noted. Then the therapist can start to look with Neil at the negative consequences of the behaviour, trying to use his phrases and only include factors that Neil agrees are relevant in order to avoid it sounding like a lecture.

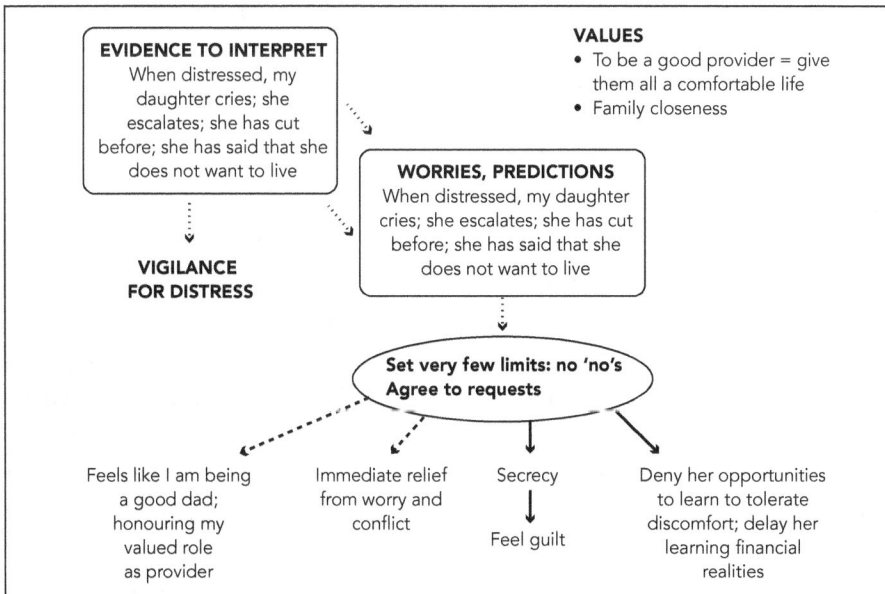

**FIGURE 4.3**
Neil's ICF sketch with motivational factors.

One potential use of this ICF sketch is to prolong a discussion with Neil about different ways to honour his value of being a father. This therapist wishes to ask Neil to weigh-up the strength of the two sides — to keep giving money or start giving nonmaterial gifts such as emotional resilience and financial responsibility and independence. (Good motivational interviewing involves the client giving voice to their concerns about the status quo and their reasons for considering uncomfortable change). This will take some time but with the right load of empathy and future-oriented questions, Neil's willingness to alter his parenting style gradually and test out some new ideas will hopefully increase.

## Important caveats

Motivational enhancement techniques, such as motivational interviewing, are rarely needed for clients who are working well in therapy. Furthermore, motivational interviewing is neither appropriate for clients who are at risk or needing more urgent intervention, nor for those who lack the cognitive sophistication to consider the advantages and disadvantages of their own choices for their longer-term future.

It is not a set of interventions that are done as a pretherapy exercise. Rather, the techniques can be woven throughout the therapy at every stage, starting with assessment, written into the formulation, then leant on more heavily whenever that client becomes ambivalent about change or manifests any type of resistance.

Finally, when it comes to motivational enhancement, timing and tone are more important than technique. Consider this question posed by a therapist of a client with a trauma-induce fear of driving, 'So, Michael, are you saying that the advantages of continuing to avoid driving a car outweigh the disadvantages of not being able to drive yourself or family members?'. This could easily be perceived as a sarcastic or bewildered challenge to the client to sort their thinking out, which would erode or even devastate the therapeutic alliance. But, depending on the timing and the tone, the client could find it validating. For instance, if the therapist had spent time highlighting and validating that client's trauma and resulting fear, and if they have acknowledged that they feel like a good father (one of his values) by staying out of perceived danger, then the above statement can be a summary of understanding that promotes reflection.

# Highlights and take-home messages

1.   All clients will experience some ambivalence towards some component of the treatment process.

2.   If the ambivalence is strong, make this the explicit object of the therapeutic conversation, rather than change-oriented interventions.

3.   CBT is mostly comprised of action-oriented interventions and yet, when a client is in a contemplative or pre-contemplative stage of change, proposing an action-oriented treatment could increase resistance and harm the TA.

4.   Align interventions with the client's stage of readiness for change for each separate behaviour or symptom.

5.   The client's willingness to engage in challenging therapeutic actions can be enhanced by known interventions, such as those taken from ACT and motivational interviewing.

# Chapter 5

# Working with all levels of cognition

> It is the mark of an educated mind to be able to entertain a
> thought without accepting it.
>
> Aristotle

C ognitive therapy is well known to encompass a range of cognitive
entities: automatic thoughts, visual imagery, predictions, comparisons, unspoken assumptions, stable beliefs and rules, core beliefs
and early maladaptive schemas. To this list we should add beliefs about
thoughts (metacognitions). We often find (sometimes with some clinical
hard work) that the cognition that is causing the most distress — the cognition that most needs to be altered — is not articulated by the client and
may lie beyond immediate awareness. This chapter is devoted to encouraging the cognitive therapist to move beyond automatic thoughts as soon
as possible and to incorporate the most potent type of cognitive entity for
each particular client's emotional disturbance.

The term 'levels of cognition' captures a stratified view of cognition and
helps the clinician to envisage why their client is having their own idiosyn-
cratic automatic thoughts, explain this to that client and incorporate the
relevant cognitions into an integrated formulation. Beck et al. (2003) have

articulated the three main layers of cognition: automatic thoughts, conditional rules or beliefs and core beliefs.

This traditional three-layered model of cognition can be extended to encompass the additional layers of metacognitions and implicit assumptions, which are described by several cognitive therapy authors (Beck, 1995; Clark & Wells, 1995; Greenberger & Padesky, 1995). These two additional layers of cognition are ubiquitous — nearly always present whenever we have 'normal' conscious automatic thoughts and yet they are often underemphasised in cognitive therapy literature. All the levels of cognition are represented in a vertical stratification model in Figure 5.1. This figure is replicated in Appendix B as a blank worksheet for use with clients. In this model we see that a person's automatic thoughts are influenced by the more stable beliefs, rules and schemas that they have internalised from their own life experiences. The lightning bolt represents how an activation of an early maladaptive schema can lead immediately and powerfully to emotions. (This is one of the few exceptions to the general rule that our emotions are

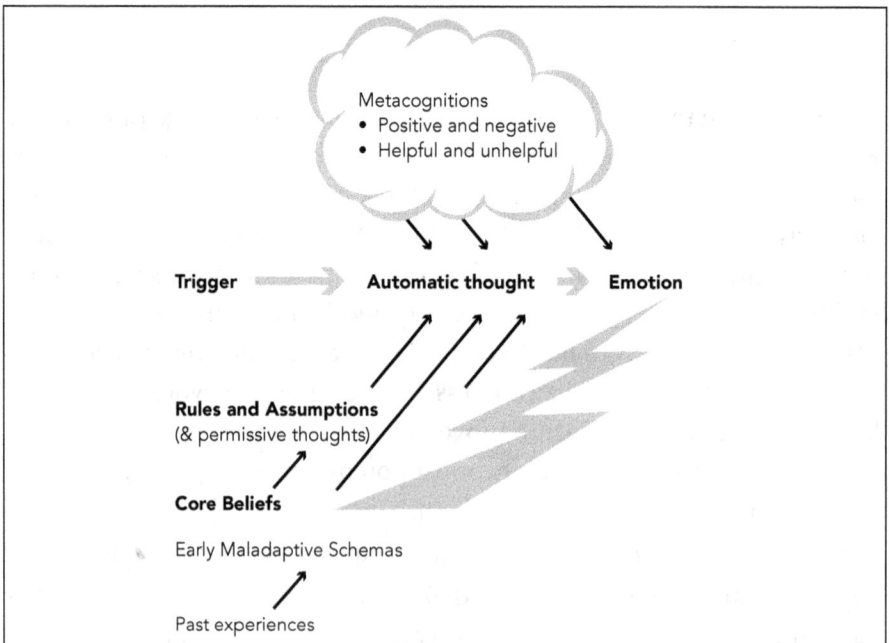

**FIGURE 5.1**
Layers cognition.

generated by our automatic thoughts; the other main exception being associative learning or classical conditioning.) The model also includes the ubiquitous thoughts, rules and beliefs that we have about our other cognitions and about our emotions — the metacognitions.

## How to help clients identify their emotions and thoughts for cognitive therapy

Before expanding on the above, it is worth taking a moment to remember that most people find it hard to learn how to use cognitive therapy for themselves. It is the therapist's task to break components down and teach a client this therapy in a useable way. These steps and subtasks include: identifying and naming a problematic emotion, identifying the relevant automatic thought, and then doing some sort of manoeuvre with the relevant cognition to alter the resultant emotion. As therapists, we spend a lot of time on the last step, helping clients dispute, redefine, correct errors, seek evidence, test predictions or defuse and ignore. All these manoeuvres depend on whether the client can access the cognitive element that most needs altering. This can often be hard. Indeed, the longer a therapist employs cognitive therapy, the more she or he is likely to take for granted the initial steps that clients find so hard — identifying which cognition actually needs challenging.

Our exemplar cases can illustrate these themes. When the cognitive model was first introduced to Neil (who presented with depression), he said that his thoughts were not the problem. Instead, he felt that the problem was the decisions he had made and how his family behaved. Amanda (with panic disorder) noted in her cognitive monitoring thoughts like, 'I have to get out of here', 'I hate this', and 'I'm feeling faint'. She said that she couldn't challenge them because she DOES hate anxiety and she DID feel faint. In each case the therapist's role is to help the client identify the thoughts that need to be challenged. This starts with helping clients to identify their automatic thoughts — often harder then we assume. The central point, however, is that most cognitive restructuring is done at levels other than automatic thoughts.

We can start with helping clients to identify their automatic thoughts, which is harder than we often assume. Unless assisted with careful exercises (not just verbal instruction) from the therapist, the typical client will find it hard to notice their thoughts and isolate the ones to be targeted in their cognitive disputation or defusion.

## Accessing automatic thoughts

> The skill of learning to identify automatic thoughts is analogous to learning any other skill. Some patients (and therapists) catch on quite quickly. Others need much more guidance and practice. (Beck 1995; p. 80)

The clinical repertoire offers many options to elicit the cognitions responsible for causing distress and dysfunction. These include *direct questions* to the client such as, *'In a typical day, how many times do you think you dwell on or think over a past decision you have made?'*, or *'When you start feeling faint, what are the biggest fears that you have about what could happen next?'*. Setting a homework task of *monitoring* the thoughts that precede problematic emotions can also be helpful. But this assumes that the client knows what to look for.

Some of the more efficient and effective ways to help clients access their cognitions are experiential exercises within the session, led by the therapist. Adrian Wells has enumerated several of these and his 2005 article on detached mindfulness and cognitive therapy techniques is highly recommended. Wells highlights the role of what he called detached mindfulness (DM) as a learnable cognitive state that enables the client to become aware of their thoughts more readily and to regard them as an observer. This allows the person to avoid automatic fusion with their thoughts; that is, to avoid regarding them as fact or reality without question. He defines DM as 'a state of awareness of internal events, without responding to them with sustained evaluation, attempts to control or suppress them, or respond to them behaviourally' (Wells, 2005; p. 340).

One of his recommended techniques, for instance, is to take a walk with your client instructing them to notice things in their *external* environment as the curious observer and simultaneously notice things in their *internal* environment as the detached observer. This takes some guiding prompts as you walk together. The clinician then enquires about their experience and what this means for their future relationship with their thoughts, especially those relating to their problematic situations.

A variation of this guided awareness process involves staying in the consultation room and anchoring the client's attention to their breath, with some brief instructions for mindful breathing:

*Bring your attention to your breath; you do not have to change your breathing or breathe in any special way; just watch the process of your breath coming in and out; trying to keep 100% of your attention on each part of each breath; it is inevitable that your mind will wander in the next few minutes — when it does that, make a note of it and gently guide your attention back to your breath.*

If clients find their breathing a poor anchor (e.g., those with panic disorder or a respiratory condition), then focusing on sensations in the hands can suffice. Then give further instructions as follows:

*Soon, I will say out aloud a few words or phrases. You do not have to do anything except keep us much attention on your breath as you can — do not try to think about the words or phrases. Your mind might respond automatically to the words. If this happens, make a note of that and then bring as much of your attention as you can back to the next breath.*

Five or six verbal stimuli are used and are presented roughly every 15 or 20 seconds and you can repeat some of the instructions if you feel necessary (e.g., 'observing how your mind responds to the words and giving yourself permission to guide your attention back to your breath). The words and phrases the therapist chooses are a mixture of neutral, negative and positive. In Amanda's case, these might be *beach* (positive), *alone* (negative), *garden* (neutral), *pillow* (neutral-positive), *fainting* (negative).

The post-exercise discussion is crucial to aid the cognitive therapy process. Typical questions to start with may include:

*Tell me about what you noticed?*

*What thoughts or images came to mind in response to word X or phrase Y?*

*Tell me ... did you have those thoughts; I mean, did **you** try to have those responses — or did **your mind** do it automatically?*

*What emotions came up for you attached to those automatic thoughts and images?*

*What was it like for you to bring your attention back to your breath?*

Take further time to explore your client's individual responses about their experience, with the goal of educating them about the role of cognition in their emotional difficulties and with a view to increasing cognitive flexibility.

An experiential exercise can be a better way to introduce the cognitive model to a new client. The aim of these exercises include helping the client to 'get' fundamental principles of the cognitive model of emotions. The fundamentals include:

- The mind can produce memories, thoughts, visual images, comparisons, predictions about the future, wishful ruminating on the past, statements about ourselves and so on and so on. These are all examples of what we call 'cognitions'.

- Most of our cognitions are automatic in nature; our mind produces them without our voluntary control.

- Some of these cognitions can produce emotions. In fact, nearly all our emotions arise from our *cognitions* about a thing, not that thing itself.

- The cognitions that our mind produces are not always relevant to us now and not necessarily helpful or accurate.

- Which means that we can decide how much attention we pay to our thoughts and we have the option of examining the cognitions objectively to determine if they are indeed helpful and accurate, and whether they are relevant to our life goals and priorities.

# Hot cognitions

Most moments of increased distress are accompanied by a stream of thoughts, predictions, assumptions, images and so on. The client may notice and record one or two thoughts but they may miss unstated rules or assumptions (see next section) or they may miss the single cognition that is causing the most distress, which we can call the 'hot cognition'. Hot cognitions are affectively loaded and important because they drive emotional distress and will impact the therapy process itself. Affective changes within session also serve golden opportunities to access cognitions — especially 'hot cognitions' (Beck, 1995). Whenever some affective change, even quite subtle, is noticed in your client, it is nearly always worth some session-time to enquire about it with questions such as:

> *What might have come up for you just then?*

> *Can you take a moment to sit with that emotion; can you name it? Is it familiar?*

> *Where does it sit in your body?*

> *Do you notice any urges associated with that feeling — such as to change the topic or another form of automatic avoidance?*

# Implicit assumptions

With every thought, there is additional cognitive material that goes unspoken. It is crucial that the therapist is alert to these implicit assumptions and helps the client perceive them. It is these assumptions or rules that often need to be challenged. All cognitive therapists are familiar with dealing with this layer of cognition (the hidden assumption). We use Socratic questioning to reveal the assumptions through a therapeutic exploration. For instance, consider the client with social anxiety who reports the cognition, *'I hate the social morning-tea meetings at work, I always start to sweat and embarrass myself'*. The therapist might wish to ask questions such as:

> *What exactly do you mean by 'embarrass' yourself — what actually happens?*, or

*Do you have an accurate assessment of what percentage of the time you perspire so that people notice?*, or

*How sure are you that people notice the sweating — can you recall evidence, such as people pointing it out?*', and

*And if someone did notice you perspiring, do you know accurately what each different individual might or might not think about that observation?*, and

*What sort of person in your workplace might change their opinion of you or judge you globally if they did notice you sweating?*

Such questions, posed within a tone of validating their discomfort and involving the client in the process of collaborative inquiry, are designed to reveal the following assumptions:

- People are looking at me a lot at these events and are focused on me enough to notice minor details.

- When I sweat, people will notice.

- All people are judgemental, and all people think the same — they are very likely to all form the same thoughts as each other about a person who perspires indoors.

- People who notice will jump to a negative conclusion about me.

- All their other interactions with me, and impressions that they have formed over the past two years, will be erased by the one sweating event.

- That would be terrible and there is nothing I can do about it.

- In the face of a fear, I should stay away.

The key point is that, in addition to using Socratic questioning in a session, the therapist can teach the client to consciously seek the unspoken assumptions that need to be challenged between sessions. This can be done by altering a cognitive monitoring form to include a column for 'sneaky assumptions' or 'unspoken hot cognition'. Some examples are illustrated later in this chapter once we have examined the other layers of cognition.

Appendix C provides an example of a client worksheet in which they are required to notice the hidden assumptions embedded in others' automatic thoughts and then leaves some space for targeted self-monitoring of their own.

## Metacognitions

In a nutshell, metacognitions are beliefs about our cognitions or our emotions, and they are ubiquitous. For every cognition, we have one or more beliefs, assumptions or rules about that cognition — it is natural that we have thoughts about our thoughts. The most common metacognition about any thought is along the lines of: 'This is a reasonable and helpful way to think'. It goes unspoken. It's more a 'sense' than a conscious thought; but it means we tend to be wedded to our thoughts as they occur in the stream of consciousness. The learnable alternative that we strive for in cognitive therapy is a form of cognitive flexibility and capacity for observing our thoughts and feelings with an appropriate level of detachment and scepticism. This is why we teach our clients maxims such as 'a thought is just a thought' and 'feelings are not facts'.

With certain types of emotional distress or psychopathology, there are more distinct metacognitions that need to be identified and possibly held up to the light for disputation and reconstructing. Adrian Wells (2006) has contributed more in this area than any other clinician and his work on worry, other anxiety disorders and the eating disorders is worth reading. Many metacognitions actively support the unhelpful thought in question or prevent the owner of those thoughts from changing or challenging them, such as 'it is not safe to think differently' or 'you are not allowed / do not deserve to feel any different to this'. Standard cognitive therapy cannot proceed and motivation for therapy stalls while these go unchallenged.

## Core beliefs

Core beliefs are stable cognitive constructs that pertain to the self, others or the world. It is important to take time early in the process of cognitive therapy to help the client appreciate what their own relevant beliefs, rules and early maladaptive schemas might be. Like automatic thoughts, these can also be illustrated with some experiential work within session. One way to introduce the idea of stable beliefs is to ask the client if they ever need consciously to remind themselves that stealing is wrong when they are shopping. When they respond in the negative, you can discuss, "I assume that you hold the belief that 'stealing is wrong' and this is a belief that guides your behaviour all the time, yet you do not think it consciously. We have hundreds of beliefs and rules that sit in our mind guiding our behaviours and feelings and we never say them out aloud and so we never question or dispute them. Thankfully, most of our core beliefs are helpful — but if there was an emotionally damaging belief amongst them, you would still act on it without articulating or questioning it". The client's rules and core beliefs could then be explored.

A generic version of these layers is presented above in Figure 5.1, and some individual examples are presented later in the chapter.

One of the chief ways to access core beliefs is through the 'downward arrow technique' that involves identifying an automatic thought and its associated emotion and asking a series of repeated questions on the two major themes of (a) *What would be the worst thing about that?*, and (b) *What would that say about you as a person or say about your life?*. It is also possible to speculate collaboratively with your client, which is how the therapist arrived at Monica's schema of incompetence. Another example might be a client who is terribly under-assertive in every life domain and experiences some social anxiety; the therapist can ask:

> *What core belief or personal rule do you have about yourself that would help us explain these two things?*
>
> *I am guessing that deep down you really feel like you are not as deserving as others.*
>
> *Does that sound right to you? How would you express what the rule or belief is on one sentence?*

Finally, the therapist also has access to questionnaires that assess core beliefs and early maladaptive schemas and the battery of Schema Questionnaires available from from Young's schema therapy website are widely used.

Each of the three clients that you are already familiar with have layers of cognitions sketched out in Figures 5.2, 5.3 and 5.4 following. You will see the same structure of metacognitions (thoughts about thoughts and beliefs about emotions) sitting above automatic thoughts, which are within an oval border. The unspoken assumptions are always in brackets; stable rules and beliefs are on a box: and if there are core beliefs or schemas, these are in a box with a double border. Amanda's layered cognitions are presented first in Figure 5.2 and it becomes clear that she could not effectively alter or defuse from her automatic thoughts until the relevant metacognitions and underlying, stable beliefs are articulated and evaluated. In Neil's case (Figure 5.3) we can again see the powerful role that unspoken assumptions and rules at different levels have on maintaining his rumination. Monica's layered cognitions are summarised in Figure 5.4 and the therapist would have added the core belief as the therapy progressed and the deeper levels of her fears and self-concept were collaboratively discovered.

To be clear, once they are identified, metacognitions can be managed with the same techniques as any automatic thought (questioning its usefulness, questioning its accuracy and relevance, doing an experiment to try to disprove it and so on). Many clients find it very helpful to develop a new set of adaptive metacognitions that are applicable to them, such as "it is safe and reasonable to ignore every one of my future thoughts about collapsing or going crazy when I'm panicking". These can be written out for familiarity and, once articulated, a series of strategies can help to reinforce the more adaptive metacognitions such as: (a) psychoeducation, (b) collating existing evidence, (c) monitoring and prospectively collecting new supportive evidence and (d) re-rating the degree to which the client believes those new beliefs each appointment.

Core beliefs typically take more time, careful strategy and therefore patience to alter. These strategies are not addressed in this chapter but are described thoroughly in other books. The key point is to be sure to identify them early and factor them into the formulation. The reader can turn to helpful texts for the core therapy skills with core beliefs, such as Beck (2005), Beck et al. (2003) and Young et al. (2003).

The fundamental strategies for conducting thought-challenging are not detailed in this book, given that the focus is on solving clinical challenges and obstacles. Nevertheless, a four-page client handout is provided in

My automatic perceptions of threat are accurate and helpful; a sense of not being in control is bad

If I feel anxious, then I am in danger (and it would be stupid not to act on that)

Vigilance of self

I'm not in control; I *have* to get out of here ⇨ FEAR ⇨ escape

(You are either in control or out of control)
(It is possible to go completely crazy from anxiety)

Anxiety is dangerous and ought to be avoided.
If I am not SURE that I am safe, then I should assume that I am not safe at all.

I am vulnerable to harm
Horrendous things can and do happen

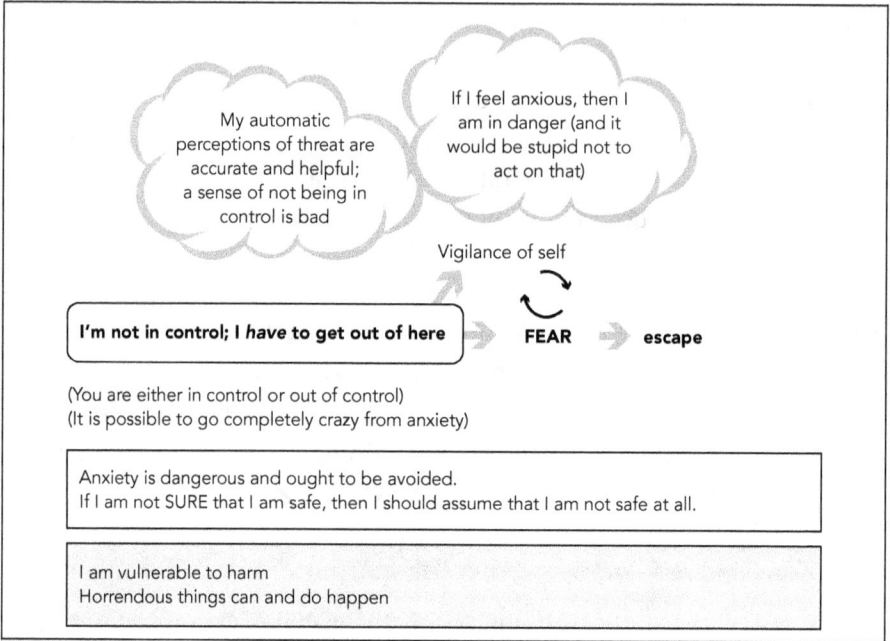

**FIGURE 5.2**
Amanda's metacognitions, unspoken assumptions, automatic thoughts, rules and core beliefs.

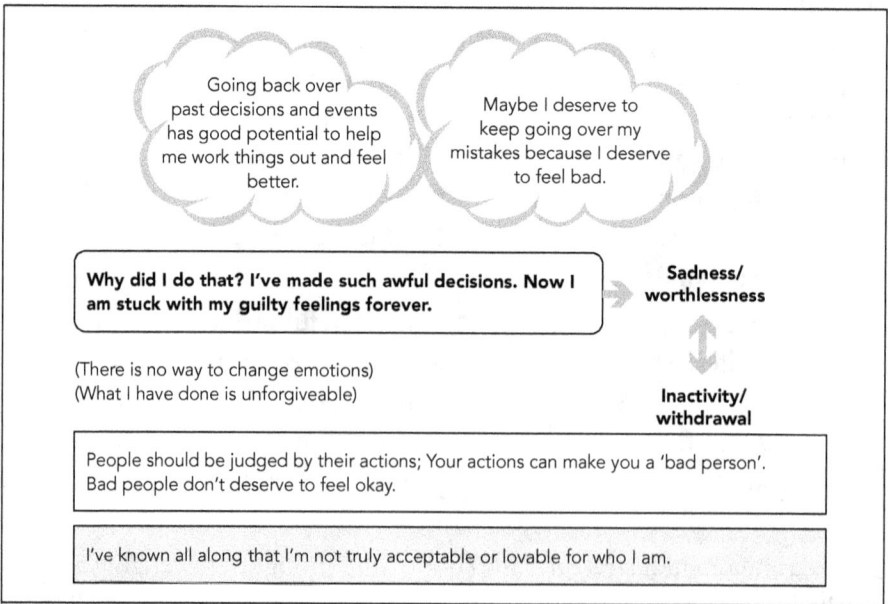

Going back over past decisions and events has good potential to help me work things out and feel better.

Maybe I deserve to keep going over my mistakes because I deserve to feel bad.

Why did I do that? I've made such awful decisions. Now I am stuck with my guilty feelings forever. ⇨ Sadness/ worthlessness

⇕ Inactivity/ withdrawal

(There is no way to change emotions)
(What I have done is unforgiveable)

People should be judged by their actions; Your actions can make you a 'bad person'. Bad people don't deserve to feel okay.

I've known all along that I'm not truly acceptable or lovable for who I am.

**FIGURE 5.3**
Neil's layered cognitions that can be noted and targeted in therapy.

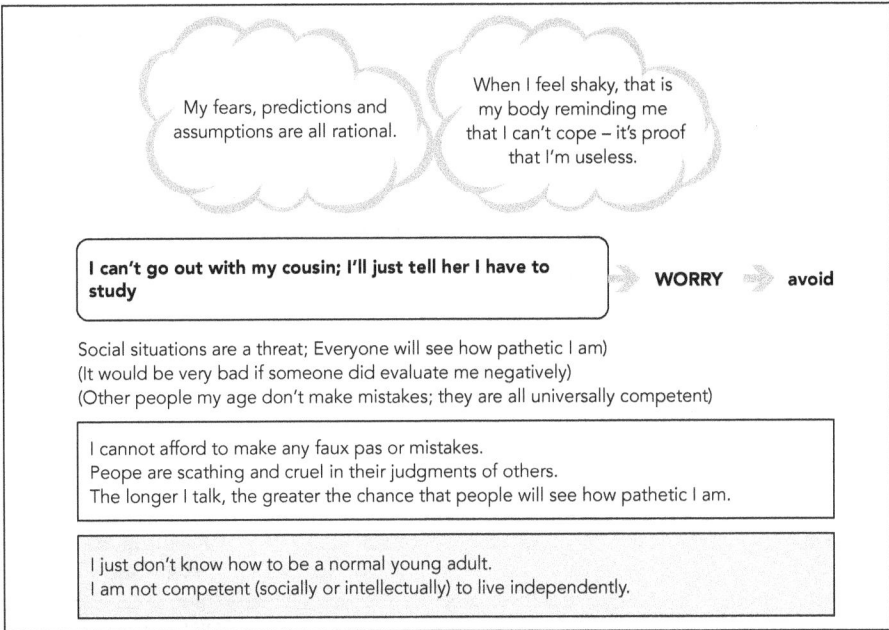

**FIGURE 5.4**
Monica's cognitions that can be noted and targeted in therapy.

Appendix D as an example of how the cognitive model and CT techniques can be introduced in writing. Such handouts should reinforce but not replace the experiential exercises and process interactions in the room with the therapist.

## Summary: Identifying the right cognition to challenge

Teaching cognitive therapy skills is hard work and one of the issues that clients find it hard to learn is which cognition they ought to challenge. Imagine the client with panic disorder who notices this automatic thought, "*I'm starting to feel shaky; I've got to get out of here*". If they try to dispute this on their own, early in therapy, how likely are they to be successful? It is desirable and possible to teach clients as quickly as possible about different types of cognition other than 'automatic thoughts'. In particular, clients do well knowing about (a) implicit assumptions – the thoughts and rules that do not get said out aloud but are known or assumed to be true, (b) 'hot cognitions' — the thought or belief that is causing the most distress, (c) metacognitions — thoughts or rules about the target thinking process and (d) stable core beliefs and rules. Table 5.1 entails a summary of these different levels of cognition, including examples of a person with panic disorder. In this client's case, the assumption could easily be *"Anxiety can turn into panic. Panic is really bad and must be avoided at all costs"*. And the hot cognition: *"I could completely lose control and embarrass myself if I panic. Someone may think I'm crazy and lock me up"*. Compared to the initial automatic thought that they recorded, they now have some content that CAN be challenged and will be emotionally HELPFUL to challenge.

**TABLE 5.1**
Summary of the main types of cognitions in the one client.

| Type of cognition | What it is | Questions to reach it | Example of the cognition |
|---|---|---|---|
| **Automatic thought** | A fleeting idea, sentence or image | What was your mind trying to tell you when you had that emotion?What phrases or images came to your mind at that time? | I'm starting to feel shaky; I've got to get out of here. |
| **Implicit assumption** | An idea or rule or assumed truth that is not consciously articulated | And why would that be bad or dangerous? What are the fears sitting behind this worry of yours? Why do other people not feel the same way as you – do they have different assumptions? | Anxiety can turn into panic. Panic is really bad and must be avoided at all costs. |
| **Hot cognition** | The thought or belief that is causing the most distress | And then – what would be so bad about that?What is the single worst thing that could possibly happen? | I could completely lose control and embarrass myself if I panic. Someone may think I'm crazy and lock me up. |
| **Metacognition** | A thought or rule about the target thinking process | What are the advantages and disadvantages of thinking this way?Do you feel that it is safe and permissible to alter this way of thinking? | It is not safe to test this out. These thoughts help me to be wary and prevent me from risking my worst fears. |
| **Core belief** | A stable, deeply held belief about the person or the world around them | What would that say about you?What is the worst thing about that? | There is something fundamentally wrong with me; I'm damaged and people are likely to see that. |

# Highlights and take-home messages

1.  Experiential exercises within a session provide a way to introduce the cognitive model to clients while also helping them to access their own automatic thoughts and feelings

2.  It is very helpful to work at multiple levels of cognition and most clients can manage to learn this form of cognitive therapy quickly

3.  The various layers of cognition can be accessed through tailoring self-monitoring between sessions, targeted psychoeducation and experiential exercises within-session

4.  Working with the unspoken assumptions is necessary, as the 'hot cognition' is rarely articulated in the automatic thought

5.  Working with metacognitions and deeper stable beliefs can help prevent and manage motivational levels that can waiver while addressing automatic thoughts.

# Chapter 6

# Creative behavioural experiments

> Experience never errs; it is only your judgements that err by promising themselves effects such as are not caused by your experiments.
>
> Leonardo da Vinci

> The trouble with most therapy is it helps you feel better. But you don't get better. You have to back it up with action, action, action.
>
> Albert Ellis

One of the most powerful agents of change is the behavioural experiment. Done well, a behavioural experiment can:

- Achieve changes in a belief (or assumption or rule), which leads to emotional change.

- Establish a new precedent, such that the client now has this behaviour in their repertoire.

- Enhance the client's self-regard and their self-efficacy for change generally.

- Strengthen the therapeutic alliance while also highlighting the active and collaborative nature of CBT.

# The nine elements of a good behavioural experiment

## 1. Rationale

There is a clear hypothesis or fear that is being tested. The client can state what they can learn, discover or disprove by doing the proposed experiment. That is, it is clear to the client how the experiment serves their own therapy goals.

## 2. Meaningful

The experiment is in line with a valued outcome for the client. The relevance to their future living is discussed, as a way to maintain motivation and willingness.

## 3. Pure discovery test

Pick one aspect to test; choose *one* thing to alter, so that accurate conclusions can be drawn about that from the planned test. Discuss what *safety behaviours* and unhealthy coping the person usually uses and how this might render the experiment ineffective. Discuss what they can and will do to cope; discuss what safety behaviours should be avoided.

## 4. Collaborative and autonomous

The client chooses whether to do the test/experiment or not. What they do and how they do it is ultimately up to them. The therapist guides and makes recommendations. The therapist can veto an experiment if they predict that it could do some harm. The client equally has the right of veto.

## 5. Adequate confidence

Use self-efficacy ratings (0 to 100). The client needs to believe that they can engage in the task. That is, they know what to do and believe they have a reasonable likelihood (e.g., 70+% self-efficacy rating) of tolerating the predicated anxiety or distress. The clinician and client both want to make as much change as possible but *always* start with something that is very likely to go well — where fear levels are mild and confidence is high. Plan for early successes, don't risk early 'failure-experiences'. It is worth erring on the side of getting a success-experience over pushing for substantial change early in therapy. Discuss and rehearse possible coping strategies for when their fears or doubts are at their highest. With time you and the client can agree to move on to more challenging experiments.

## 6. Anticipation of potential problems and challenges

Some problems cannot be anticipated but it is good to take time to collaboratively wonder what might make the experiment complicated, ambiguous or hard to complete. If the client's anxiety might become more than predicted, it would be good to have some contingencies ready. For instance, they have the option of making the experiment slightly easier, rather than choosing to desist completely. In the same vein, it may be wise to agree in advance to do the same exercise three or even five times (repeated measures data-collection yields better reliability).

## 7. Written plan and baseline observations

Write out exactly what the new goal behaviour is. Write out the client's fearful predictions or assumptions and imagery. Note current baseline functioning and responding.

## 8. Monitoring

Using the same form as the fearful predictions (previous step), the client documents what actually DID happen in the most objective format possible. See Appendix E for an example of a worksheet for a behavioural experiment.

## 9. Incorporation into therapy goals

Once any test has been done, work out with the client what was discovered. What conclusions can be drawn? What are the implications for their everyday living? The next time they are in a fearful situation, what can they think or do differently? What are the next one or two tests that make sense at this point?

Let's look at how to apply these rules of thumb to two of our three familiar case studies.

### Amanda

Amanda is a 31-year-old woman with panic disorder. Her panic attacks are characterised by an overwhelming feeling that she is going to collapse or faint and feels 'out of control'. At times, she feels sure than her heart will stop beating. Her legs 'feel like jelly' and she feels that she must sit down.

She is reluctant to do *in vivo* exposure to places that she fears, such as driving to new suburbs or going to a new café or shopping mall. Exploring the cognitive basis of this reveals that she is scared of what can happen to her when she gets anxious and this fear has persisted despite very clear repeated psychoeducation from the therapist already. The therapist decides to help her to disprove her fears about anxiety through behavioural experimentation.

1. **Explain the rationale.** The goal is to reduce Angela's fear of her own anxiety response and this requires the deliberate, prolonged and repeated exposure to sensations in her body that she associates with anxiety. Wonder together exactly how an experiment is going to lessen her fear. There needs to be a prediction or belief to test out and you may wish to discuss how many times to run the same experiment to draw sound conclusions:

   *Will one instance of reassuring evidence change your mind?*

   *What if it does not go perfectly, would you be willing to do it several times to test it out further?*

2. **Articulate specific fears that can be targeted.** Amanda expressed her beliefs regarding her own anxiety response:

   • *I really could collapse or faint and then injure myself (it feels so real; how can I not faint?),* and

   • *If the anxiety reaches its peak, I might never regain control.*

   • *I could lose my ability to think or talk; I will embarrass myself and I could end up in a psychiatric hospital long term.*

3. **Attend to the relationship.** Take time to validate how terrifying these thoughts are. Clients tend to be more trusting and flexible with their therapeutic tasks if they feel that their distress and fears have been acknowledged and understood. It is tempting to move straight to education, coaching in thought-challenging or a behavioural experiment. Let Amanda know that you do not share her fears at all

but that you can see why she is so reluctant to have anxiety. The following might help:

*Your fears include injury, humiliation and possibly losing control of your whole person. That is super scary; no wonder you spend a lot of energy and stress making sure that you never get too anxious. That makes sense to me now.*

4. **Attend to motivation.** Briefly enhance her motivation to address these fears and internalise responsibility for her own outcomes. Some questions at this point like the following could prove helpful:

*The outcomes you fear are indeed terrifying; but if there was a safe way to test out the likelihood of your fears, would you be willing to try that?*

*Any such experiment would make you feel more scared temporarily, so why would you be willing to do that? What is so important about the way you want to live your life in the future that means you would be willing to provoke your fears?*

5. **Fear hierarchy.** Generate a list of situations together that cause her anxiety and therefore wants to avoid. After ranking them for difficulty, the collaborative list may look like this:

   • Running up 3 flights of stairs (to induce shortness of breath, racing heart and feeling hot)

   • Deliberate hyperventilation (to induce feeling clammy and light-headed)

   • Spinning around until feeling dizzy (to induce feeling shaky and unsteady and faint)

   • Watching a scary movie with: someone; on my own; on my own at night) (to induce a fear response)

   • Imagining a future panic attack (to induce fear)

   • Recalling a past bad panic attack (to induce fear)

6. **Anticipate difficulties and how to manage them.** Amanda is told that she is in control of the process — she gets to stop or get to safety

whenever she wants. She is reminded, though, that each time she tolerates her anxiety longer than she wants, it is a powerful opportunity to disprove her fears and be liberated from them for the rest of her life. She is encouraged to imagine herself getting anxious and choosing to sit with that uncertainty and discomfort. She is encouraged to use healthy coping strategies and to avoid safety behaviours that would undermine the effectiveness of the test. A healthy coping strategy might be to recall times when she did not faint or recall the psychoeducation that she has been given. Rehearse with Angela how she will resist the urge to sit down when feeling light-headed, dizzy and shaky.

7. **Get going.** The therapist can set the tone of these experiments. The anxious client like Amanda will be helped by doing it efficiently and with a fairly matter-of-fact tone (neither dismissive of the level of challenge, nor dwelling too much on how scary it is). It is also helpful to do the activities together and many clients will be emboldened when they see their therapist modelling the feared actions with them or just before them.

8. **Reflection.** After the experiment has been conducted, congratulate Amanda on her effort. Encourage her to reflect on what she was pleased with. Discuss how you both felt, assuming you did the experiment together. Discuss what evidence was gathered. In Amanda's case, the most likely outcome would be that she would experience some physic al sensations, then a wave of intense anxiety, which will then decrease gradually. Discuss how this fits with the psychoeducation that she has been provided and with what other people tend to believe. What are the implications for (a) the next experiment that could be done and (b) when she next starts to feel anxious? Ask Amanda if she can now give herself permission to think differently about her fears in the future and discuss why many people with panic disorder do get contradictory evidence but without it leading to a sense of safety.

### Neil

Neil is a 58-year-old man requesting help for his depression. He feels trapped in the weekly financial support of one of his two daughters, who is depressed herself and does not work. She has engaged in some suicidal gestures before (an overdose of her antidepressants, after which she called him) and she talks of suicide from time to time when upset. He pays her rent, a living allowance and a personal grooming allowance. He is terrified that she will get more depressed and kill herself is she is stressed about money or if he denies a request. But his other daughter is losing respect for him, he is lying about the money to his wife and he is sure that he will run out of money for his own retirement.

1. **Explain the rationale.** The goal is to disprove Neil's intense fear that his daughter will suicide if he sets some reasonable limits around money. An interim goal would be to establish a set of methods to test out this fear and then find out which Neil would consider 'safe enough' to attempt.

2. **Articulate specific fears that can be targeted.** Neil worked out with his therapist that the most relevant belief was worded thus:

   - *My daughter is quite likely to get hysterically distressed when I tell her that her allowances need to be reduced and then there is a good chance that she will want to kill herself again (and she will make a serious attempt, and she won't get help and she could die).*

3. **Attend to the relationship.** Empathise with how a responsible and anxious a father would feel if he thought his daughter might want to end her own life. Then build up a shared understanding about how he has become so stuck in this financial and emotional dependent trap by highlighting that he is trying to honour his values around being a good father. Let him know that he has been doing the best job he possibly can in a difficult situation — one that nobody could judge unless they have been in exactly the same boat.

4. **Attend to motivation.** Given that Neil feels paralysed by fear and he has been unable to change these behaviours for years, his readiness for change will need considerable attention to get him to the point of doing an experiment. A therapist could use any combination of these following approaches:

   - Having identified with how much value he places on being a good, caring father, then ask a series of Socratic questions designed to help him redefine 'good parenting' as a process that results in adult children being independent and emotionally robust.

- Then it is a small step away to discuss whether he could see setting limits as another manifestation of being a good parent.

- Discuss how his daughter might actually benefit from a gentle and gradual reduction in the unchecked financial support she is afforded.

- Ask him to list five other long-term advantages of setting limits on his daughter's profligate spending, apart from him then being released from his fear and her learning to be more self-reliant and responsible as a young adult. The therapist might prompt to get at points such as: he might then be able to have a better relationship with his other daughter; he can have a better relationship with the depressed daughter — a relationship no longer built on money and fear but on other interactions; he would not feel that his value of honesty is compromised, as he would have less to lie about; he would have more money for all his family.

- Ask him to consider the harm to her that may inadvertently occur if he cannot find a way to broach the topic of limits. Start Socratic and contribute with suggestions that other parents might consider.

5. **Fear hierarchy**. Brainstorm a large number of possible ways to broach the topic of money with his daughter, such that there is a gradient of fear and then he could be asked to select the option that would make him the least afraid. These options might include:

- Have a general discussion that **maybe** at **some point** her allowance would **probably** decrease.

- Wait until there is an extra request for money (not the usual weekly allowance) and decline that — do not yet bring up the idea that there will be a permanent reduction in monies.

- Giving her two or four months' notice of any changes in regular allowance.

- Telling her that for family financial reasons he needs to reduce her allowance by 10% every month over six months.

- Have someone else present at the time of the conversation (or not).

Ultimately, ask Neil if there is *any* conversation that he would be willing to have with her.

6. **Anticipate difficulties and how to manage them.** It might be helpful to reiterate that, in Neil's anxious mind, this is literally a life-or-death situation and he will be very scared. His daughter has a history of mentioning suicide to alter people's behaviour, including his. This can be discussed candidly, given that a strong therapeutic alliance has been established. How will Neil feel if she mentions distress or wanting to die? Is he aware of ways to get her help other than money, such as a referral to a mental health professional?

The therapist can role-play with Neil how he can respond to her declarations of distress and thoughts about dying. This would include how to organise swift access to hospital-based care in the event that she became unsafe. It would also be helpful to decide in advance how to manage his worry after the conversation, as that is when Neil may experience his highest worry. Finally, decide together what a 'good outcome' could be. For instance, the therapist would want to suggest that if Neil initiates the conversation, feels anxious and guilty during the conversation and his daughter cries and employs a degree of emotional persuasion — then that could still be a good outcome. He has tried a new behaviour and his worst fears were not realised — it just felt really awful.

7. **Get going.** Some action steps could be undertaken in a consultation. It is also possible to set a homework task for Neil to write up a plan, including mode and the exact timing of the communication with his daughter.

8. **Reflection.** If he goes ahead, then the reflection on the conversation will be crucial. Unlike most behavioural experiments, it is unlikely in this case that the therapist will be present to help collate evidence and moderate the experience. There is a reasonable likelihood also that Neil will experience anxiety before and after the conversation.

As already noted above, some careful anticipation of this is warranted, as will be a discussion about what he learned about his fears and his coping strategies.

# Troubleshooting with behavioural experiments

## What if the client does not want to do experiments?

The therapist's first tasks in this circumstance are to understand the basis of this reluctance and then convey that empathic comprehension to the client. It is then possible to target the client's fears through classic cognitive therapy procedures (such as, information-provision, Socratic questioning or establishing a much smaller test). The therapist will also seek to highlight the discrepancy between their client's (understandable) avoidance choices and their future goals. This can be done by asking questions about what they would love to do in life if not held back by this anxiety; or perhaps exploring the top five personal costs of accommodating this fear into their life. Read back over Chapter 4 for more detailed suggestions. Then, finally, use a visual analogue scale of confidence to find out what they think they feel capable, suggesting a range of relatively easy challenges to start with.

## What if the therapist is hesitant to do a behavioural experiment?

Behavioural experiments are perhaps the single most powerful tool in our kit as cognitive therapists. Take some time to identify the basis for your hesitation. Is there a doubt about the necessity of such an intervention? A therapist may fear how the client will cope — worry worry that excessive client distress will set the client back or harm the therapeutic alliance. We need to examine our own beliefs about client distress levels. A well-planned and constructed experiment can avoid the worst outcomes. Clients do experience some emotional distress in some experiments. Often the primary or secondary target of a useful experiment is to discover that the distress is tolerable and passes without any desperate coping efforts. Many argue strongly that emotional distress in a therapy session is actually helpful in many ways. A client may learn that (a) their fears do not come true, (b) all feelings pass without harm, (c) that others can tolerate their distress, (d) that we cannot overcome an anxiety disorder without being willing to feel fear, (e) that we cannot move towards some of our values in life without choosing some discomfort, and (f) that temporary discomfort and distress saves us from longer-term greater suffering. It is typically the case that experiencing some distress within a session, where this can be acknowledged and contained, aids the therapeutic alliance and does not harm it.

Several authors have provided helpful exposition on why clinicians do not employ interventions of known effectiveness (Lilienfeld et al., 2013; Waller, 2009, 2016; Waller & Turner, 2016). All therapists invested in getting optimal outcomes for their clients are well advised to consider these issues and read such articles. As therapists, there are several ways to reduce our own worries or cautions. These include discussing in supervision, disputing anxious predictions and conducting a well-planned formal behavioural experiment of our own (in this case, about experiments).

## What if a well-planned experiment goes wrong?
All experienced cognitive therapists have had some surprises when doing experiments with clients. We can prepare ourselves and the clients for such occurrences. The main contingency responses lie within the experimental method. At the planning stage, the therapist might anticipate unpredicted and unwanted outcomes and make suggestions accordingly, such as to use repeated measures (agree to do the same experiment three or five times before starting). In the aftermath of an unwanted or unpredicted outcome, it is important to debrief and decatastrophise as quickly as possible. It may be possible to highlight ALL the evidence that was collected in the experiment, as some will be neutral, some helpful and some unhelpful. But the client may focus exclusively on one aspect — the danger cues. We can ask the client what other factors (variables in the experiment) were relevant here that need to be taken into account. If the issue was that the client found the experiment too anxiety provoking, then (a) take time to discuss what they were thinking or focusing on to cause such distress and coach in cognitive therapy skills and (b) suggest a new variation that will be considerably easier. It is advisable to do this immediately so the session concludes with a success experience.

## What if a fear is not readily testable?
Many fears are not easily tested in a behavioural experiment. Notorious examples include when the feared consequences are a long way into the future (like an OCD fear in which a failure to perform a ritual could cause

illness or death several months hence) or when the fear is not measurable (such as fear of negative evaluation in the form of a private opinion held by another person). In each case, it may still be worthwhile to discuss the role of behavioural experimentation with the client. The idea and the *spirit* of collaborative empiricism can play a role outside the actual experiments themselves. If the client appreciates the rationale for experimentation with their fears, then they may grab an opportunity when it arises. It may also be possible to do a partial experiment. For instance, in the case of fear of negative evaluation (where you will never know for sure what a person is thinking) it is possible to ask the client to define what behaviours they would observe if the other person did judge them negatively, such as staring, grimacing or treating them differently.

The client can also use an *Observational* experiment instead of the more common *Active* experiments (Rouf, Fennel, Westbrook, Cooper, & Bennet-Levy, 2004). This would involve systematically monitoring others engaging in normal behaviours that the client feels are unsafe and noting outcomes. This could take 10 minutes (for someone with social phobia to observe people in retail situations), or an hour (for someone with PTSD to observe how safe people are walking down to street if they are not being vigilant for assault) or three weeks (in the case of someone with OCD where the fear is of catching a viral infection in the office unless specific precautions are taken).

# Highlights and take-home messages

1. Behavioural experiments are one of the more powerful tools to achieve cognitive, emotional and behavioural changes.

2. Be absolutely clear about what is being tested and discovered.

3. Be attentive to the narrow therapeutic window and start with an easy grade of fear in order to get a success-experience.

4. Experiments are most likely to work well when done within a consultation with the therapist present. Be creative and leave the consulting room if needs be.

5. Examine your own reasons (your beliefs, assumptions, predictions, etc.) for not doing more behavioural experiments with clients.

# Chapter 7

# Getting on track and staying on track: Avoiding therapeutic drift

> Our tendency to drift away from evidence-based practice is the product of a range of very human experiences and characteristics. These factors mean that we engage in safety behaviours.
>
> Waller & Turner (2016)

The term 'staying on track' implies that, based on your formulation, a planned pathway of certain interventions will be delivered in a meaningful sequence over several sessions. It also refers to the crucial tradition in CBT of adhering to a strategic treatment plan for one or two presenting issues. If we chip away at the hardest nut consistently enough for long enough, in a collaborative alliance with our client, then it will crack. If we keep trying different approaches or pick a different nut every few weeks, then we will crack none.

The term 'therapist drift' traditionally refers to the way a therapist ceases to employ treatment of documented effectiveness. This is a serious (and arguably an ethical) issue. In this chapter the slightly different term 'therapeutic drift' refers more to the tendency to waiver from generating outcomes in a time-limited way.

## Responsibility

It is the *therapist's* responsibility to prevent either type of drift; we cannot expect a client to anticipate it happening, nor know how to pull the therapy back into the most effective line. Indeed, we ought to understand that most clients will inadvertently instigate some therapeutic drift for common reasons such as avoidance of unpleasant emotions or the immediacy-effect of current problems.

An inventory of self-assessment questions for this responsibility might include:

- How often have your clients wanted to change the main focus of therapy or add new presenting concerns after the initial assessment?

- If so, has this altered the concentration of the 'dose' of treatment that you can deliver for the first presenting problem that they want help with?

- What does the literature say about the most effective treatment for the problems that you commonly treat? To what degree do you employ those methods?

- Have you ever treated a condition with the skill-set that you possess already rather than the treatment that has the most evidence?

- What are your reasons for not using the treatment with the most effective evidence-base, and are they valid?

- At what point should we tell our clients that we are actually not using the treatment that has the most evidence for their condition and obtain fresh consent to proceed with a treatment that could be considered alternative?

- Should a clinician be required to use only one treatment method or follow only one theoretical model for a given client because it has more support than other approaches thus far?

## Staying on track with homework

Therapy exercises between consultations constitute one of the defining features of CBT. The setting and the completing of between-session tasks have been found to be associated with more effective treatments (Kazantzis, Deane & Ronan, 2000). The setting of homework by the therapist and its completion by the client is therefore crucial in staying on track and producing better outcomes.

The 'dose' of CBT that the client receives will alter the outcome that the client obtains and that *dose* is affected by variables associated with the therapist, the client and the task itself. The therapist has greater influence over the task factors and therapist factors, as they affect homework compliance (Tompkins, 2006). A prescribed task needs to be clearly relevant to the client, have a sound rationale and be within the client's capacities to complete. The therapist needs to discuss exactly how and when to do this task and anticipate motivational hurdles as well as potential practical and environmental obstacles. The task needs to be clear and written down, so there's no misinterpretation or reliance on memory. A method for recording or monitoring efforts and outcomes must also be decided and arranged. Remember that a collaborative decision to set this particular homework increases ownership and compliance.

A helpful checklist of therapist-variables includes:

- Take some time to ask the client what their costs and concerns of doing the exercise might be, so that these can be acknowledged and maybe resolved.

- Have you been clear? Can the client repeat what they are to do and how it serves their treatment goals?

- Ask the client to write out what the agreed homework task is. This serves as a check-point to be sure that they have understood and can recall it, while also encouraging them to own the task.

- Ask the client to state why they would be willing to spend time and generate discomfort for this exercise (eliciting the client's own reasons for change-behaviours is a motivational interviewing technique; see Chapter 4).

- Check that their self-efficacy for doing this is at least 70% and alter the exercise if not.

- Allocate a suitable amount of time for reviewing homework at the next session.

Appendix F is an example of an end-of-session list of questions that the client completes, guided by the therapist. It includes a space for the client to write their understanding of the 'homework' tasks, as well as self-monitoring and goals until next consultation. This particular sheet also includes three of the four questions from Miller et al.'s (2003) Session Rating Scale (which the therapist does not guide but does discuss).

The TA can be prioritised through the homework prescription and especially upon reviewing the homework at the next session. If homework is incomplete or incorrect, praise the effort and discuss what *has* been done — then ask permission to explore how it could be done more thoroughly or more closely aligned with the actual rationale. If not done at all, then this needs to be discussed. It may help to increase therapeutic allegiance and future compliance if the therapist can create a tolerable degree of tension by asking a series of questions; for example:

> *What factors affected your ability or willingness to do the homework?*

> *What implications does this have for how we run today's session?*

> *Let's both be more careful when we set the homework at the end of today's session.*

If the therapist senses that the client is feeling too chastised, it is possible to check in and soothe the TA; for example:

> *Do you mind me asking these questions?*

> *We both want the same thing, which is the best outcome for you and so I'm keen to chat openly about the homework — does that feel okay with you?*

If the homework is done well, then generous and descriptive praise is due; for example:

*I can see that you put quite a bit of time into this — I'm impressed and I'm confident that it'll help you get some good results;* and

*I like the way that you ...*

*What factors contributed to you making that good effort with the agreed homework task?*

## How does therapeutic drift occur?

Be alert to several slippery slopes. Examples include:

- Drifting away from one clear therapeutic approach that is grounded in a coherent theoretical model supported by evidence. This type of drift could occur because the client does not initially respond positively to a chosen treatment. Or perhaps the therapist feels that their clinical judgement is superior to the published evidence-based treatments available in the literature. It also sometimes occurs due to lack of education and awareness on the part of the therapist of what the most effective treatments entail. As a result, the treatment is likely to become dilute and lose efficacy.

- Other therapists are aware of an effective treatment but are disinclined to use it regardless. Lilienfeld et al. (2013) have outlined a multitude of reasons why therapists elect not to use evidence-based and manualised treatments, as discussed earlier in this book. Without repeating that discussion here, it is worth noting that a meta-analysis has shown that manualised therapy protocols tend to be more effective than clinical judgement (Grove et al., 2000). What's more, effectiveness of clinical judgement does not increase with duration of experience; Shapiro and Shapiro (1982) famously found that therapists can tend to become less effective with years beyond graduating.

- Therapists' emotions, if not noticed or managed well, are a common source of drift. A therapist will inevitably have emotional reactions within a consultation and these reactions need to be managed. For instance, it is known that clinicians who cannot tolerate distress in their client with post-traumatic stress elect not to use effective treatments

(Deacon & Farrell, 2013). Similarly, the greater the anxiety in clinicians treating eating disorders, the less likely they were to suggest known CBT interventions (Waller, 2016). Waller and Turner (2016) highlight many points in their article on therapist drift, especially emotional avoidance in the therapist:

> Our concerns about challenging or distressing our patients through the use of behavioural or cognitive change can result in our engaging in clinician safety behaviours — not pushing patients to change, so that our self-identity as positive characters in their lives is not threatened. (p. 131).

- The therapist has trouble reserving time for one or two presenting issues. Clients may raise multiple different presenting problems that shift in terms of priority over time. For instance, there may be a series of different crises that demand attention most sessions — and after several appointments there has been no change in the main presenting concern. The result is that the client and therapist make no progress over time in achieving lasting change on any one issue. The client may ultimately feel that the therapy seems directionless and is not meeting their initial expectations (even if it was *they* who wanted to discuss a range of stressors).

- The client lacks willingness to work hard on one or more goals but instead is more content to attend for supportive counselling. The result is that they will not achieve much emotional or behavioural change over time. At worst, they will come to rely on appointments to meet their emotional or even social needs.

The following brief clinical guidance may be of use to inoculate from therapeutic drift or to bring it back on track swiftly if you discover that the drift has already started to occur. The discussion starts with *primary prevention* (how to avoid drift from occurring in the first place) and then addresses *secondary prevention* (once noticed, how to avoid it deepening or becoming more problematic).

## Preventative strategies

These strategies include:

- Plan ahead. Anticipate drift with your clients with a pre-emptive conversation. This can include the warning that you may perceive a need to interrupt at some points and redirect the conversation.

- Use some formal psychoeducation about the nature of effective therapy. We often do this with our clients and a CB therapist uses informal approaches (shaping behaviours over time and role-modelling) and formal induction (written statements) to 'socialise' the client to the therapy process. An example of a client information sheet is provided in the Appendix G, titled 'The seven pillars of effective therapy'.

- Use formal reviews and 'check-ins' of treatment direction and effectiveness. These could be done, say, every five appointments. They could also be at the half-way point of every appointment, at which point you collaboratively address questions such as:

  *Are we using our time today to your best advantage?*

  *What are the chief priorities for the remainder of the session?*

  *Is any emotional avoidance creeping in?*

- Use visual prompts in session, such as your hand-drawn formulation in a highly visible place. Or write out an agenda on a sheet of paper in the room for you and the client to see.

- One approach that employs both a visual cue and a formal review is to employ an 'end-of-session summary' page. This should be in sight throughout the session and the client takes 3 to 5 minutes to complete at the end. As already noted, an example is provided in the Appendix F. After a few sessions, the therapist and client should both feel accountable to the questions routinely being asked.

- Talk explicitly with the client about the 'dose of treatment' that they are getting, perhaps using pain medication as an analogy (*'If you had a blinding migraine, would you take half of one paracetamol?'*). It is the therapist's role to explain what a 'full dose of cognitive therapy' is and to prescribe exercises between sessions accordingly. Heed Waller's (2009) advice that optimal treatment is 168-hour-a-week therapy, with one of these hours being a consultation.

- Have clinical supervision and bring your clients up in discussion. At the very least, imagine how you would present this client in supervision and then predict your supervisor's response and suggestions.

- Type up and frequently refer to a checklist of questions to help create a self-conscious accountability to staying 'on track'. Some favourite self-posed questions include:

  *What will my client be saying to their referring doctor or a family member about what treatment we are doing?*

  *If they need to see another psychologist in a year from now for the same problem, what will they tell that psychologist about the treatment methods that we used?*

  *This client is giving up a lot to come to treatment, so what do they deserve from me each and every session?*

  *If I had a close relative with exactly the same problem as this client, what treatment would I expect? Would I want their therapist to do their best to pick an evidence-based treatment and apply it skilfully to my loved-one; or would I be happy for them to decide on their own treatment plan and maybe change this from time to time?*

### Secondary prevention

If the therapist realises that drift has already started to occur, then potential solutions include:

- Redirect the conversation. If an ineffective 10 minutes of session time has just passed, then intervene. This may require a change of topic that can feel abrupt but we need to remind ourselves as therapists that this is not a social relationship but a professional helping relationship and so we have a licence (arguably a responsibility) to be as direct as the client can tolerate. If a client is sensitive to invalidation or feels a need to be overly thorough in their narratives, then share the dilemma with the client. That is to say, the two of you need to consider what is the lesser of two negatives — they feel interrupted or the therapy lacks direction and focused interventions.

- If it is a more significant drift (e.g., trouble keeping traction on any one goal over several sessions), then start by naming the process with the client. Reflect, without blame, that the therapy has lacked the focused intensity that is needed to achieve the changes for which they initially presented. Suggest that you and they discuss now how to manage this in all future treatment appointments. The therapist can articulate the need to preserve some time for therapy techniques and exercises that are designed to achieve change over time, while still asking the client for their opinion about their needs and expectations.

- Consider asking your client what their preference is — especially if they have been avoidant of harder session-content. Discuss alternatives to unhelpful drift. This may need one or more sessions devoted to motivational interviewing. Start with a cost–benefit analysis of continuing with the recent trend, while empathising with their reasons for drifting away from the more effective (often harder) interventions. Then reflect together if this is in line with the life that they wish for their future ('developing the discrepancy', as seen in Chapter 4).

- Bring the ICF sketch to more prominent attention in the session and discuss together what has been happening. Is there a new layer or new factor that can be written into the formulation to help both of you see what has been happening? One example may be an obsessional need for thoroughness, or a heightened need to be heard and validated? Perhaps there are social problems that cause more stress every week independent of the main presenting problem.

- You may wish to suggest that you both spend a certain number of sessions refocusing on just one therapeutic goal or sub-goal.

- Discuss termination and ask your client afresh what changes they wish to have achieved before the therapy inevitably comes to an end.

- Be willing to end therapy. While this sounds counterintuitive, it can be very powerful and enable a useful conversation (Waller, 2012). If the therapist is more invested in therapy and the outcomes than the client, then this needs to be said out aloud with the option of discontinuation if that is what the client wants. The tone with which this is stated is crucial. Often, the client then starts to argue why they do want to continue, perhaps with more realistic and honest goals. The therapist has every right to remind the client that, in order to continue, there needs to be evidence of improvement over time; safety and effectiveness are the main requirements in therapy. An analogy can be instructive if we ask a client:

*Imagine someone you love is seeing a cardiologist for a serious heart condition and, after four months, the treatment is not working. If the cardiologist at that point suggested continuing with the same treatment for another month or so, what would you think? Personally, I'd insist on them changing treatment or referring to a new cardiologist.*

Our case study of Monica, with social anxiety, could be used as an example here. She has a pattern of raising a variety of concerns (her belief that her parents think she's lazy; study and time-management issues; friendship issues; acute anxiety attacks; social anxiety; exam anxiety). On the day where a behavioural experiment was planned, she says she wants to discuss her painful feelings about an unflattering photo that a friend posted of the two of them. This is an important and potentially helpful opportunity to discuss several things. Firstly, though, if the therapist is frustrated with the avoidance or process, they need be conscious of this so they can avoid expressing that frustration in any way (many clients have a learned hyper-sensitivity to annoyance in others). The next step would be to give voice to the ambivalence about the treatment process in today's session and, if that is well received, it may be possible to generalise or discuss the trend of avoiding certain themes.

The following statements might be employed in this instance:

*Monica, I'm often happy to discuss issues that are important to you — but the more we do that, the less time we have to work on therapy tasks that will achieve the outcomes we've agreed to prioritise.*

*Why don't we take a little more time and care than we usually do to set the agenda for today's session. You wanted to add the issue of the photo to the agenda. And we are both aware that we had planned to do that behavioural experiment. What are the pros and cons of starting with the photo issue?*

*It occurs to me that one of the advantages of discussing the friend who posted the photo is that it means we don't have to do the experiment. I'd say 100% of my clients tend to get nervous and hesitant with such experiments. Would it be alright with you if we talk about the photo issue later and we start by addressing your feelings about some of the therapy exercises and, in particular, your motivational balance for trying to disprove one fear at a time through planned experiments?*

*While we are talking about this, I think we should both feel free to explore the various mixed feelings that you have about getting better generally — not just about today's planned experiment. I remind myself that in your mind you believe that you can't do things right — that you need others or you will inevitably fail miserably. So, then it makes sense in a way to stay unwell. I mean, plenty of people would feel safer if they were obviously having trouble or still seeing a psychologist. So, it's kind of inevitable that, at some point (perhaps already), your mind will have some doubts about the safety and desirability of 'getting better'.*

Throughout the summary above, the therapist is normalising and validating the idea of secondary gain from the sick role. Here are some questions for further consideration:

*What quality of TA would you need to have to be this candid with Monica?*

*Would **you** feel comfortable raising these issues with a client like Monica?*

*What doubting cognitions come to mind about raising these issues? How do you know if your doubts are accurate and helpful?*

*What costs to the therapy will remain if you do not raise these issues candidly?*

Let us conclude as the chapter started — with a 'tough-love' reminder from Waller and Turner (2016; p. 134), who state: 'the prevention of therapist drift requires intra-clinician comparison of outcomes — are we getting better or worse at getting our patients well? Using outcomes to acknowledge that some clinicians do poorly and some do better than the norm allows us to understand which clinicians might be exemplars of best practice'. As was discussed in Chapter 3 on the therapeutic alliance, there is great potential benefit for our clients if we are willing to systematically measure the outcomes that we are obtaining.

# Highlights and take-home messages

1. Therapist drift refers to when a therapist may not use or adhere to all the components of a treatment with proven effectiveness.

2. Therapeutic drift is the tendency to drop the focus from one or two clear therapy goals such that the client is less likely to achieve measurable outcomes.

3. Both types of drift are common and can be prevented through the therapist anticipating their occurrence and understanding their own contributing factors.

4. It is the therapist's responsibility to keep each session on track and keep the therapy on track in a way that is accountable to outcomes and proven treatments.

# References

Alexander, L.B., & Luborsky, L. (1986). The Penn Helping Alliance Scales. In L.S. Greenberg & W.M. Pinsof (Eds.), *Guilford Clinical Psychology and Psychotherapy series. The Psychotherapeutic Process: A Research handbook* (pp. 325–366). New York, NY: Guilford Press.

Arnow, B.A., Steidtmann, D., Blasey, C., Manber, R., Constantino, M.J., Klein, D.N., Markowitz, J.C., … Kocsis, J.H. (2013). The relationship between the therapeutic alliance and treatment outcome in two distinct psychotherapies for chronic depression. *Journal of Consulting and Clinical Psychology, 81*(4), 627–638.

Baldwin, S.A., Wampold, B.E., & Imel, Z.E. (2007). Untangling the alliance-outcome correlation: Exploring the relative importance of therapist and patient variability in the alliance. *Journal of Consulting and Clinical Psychology, 75*, 842–852.

Bandura, A. (1977). Self-efficacy: Toward a unifying theory of behavioral change. *Psychological Review, 84*(2), 191.

Barlow, D.H. & Craske, M.G. (2001). *Panic Disorder and Agoraphobia.* New York, NY: Guilford Press.

Barlow, D.H., Farchione, T.J., Bullis, J.R., Gallagher, M.W. (2017). The unified protocol for transdiagnostic treatment of emotional disorders compared with diagnosis-specific protocols for anxiety disorders: A randomized clinical trial. *JAMA Psychiatry. 74*(9), 875–884. doi:10.1001/jamapsychiatry.2017.2164

Beck, A.T., Freeman, A., Davis, D., & Associates (2003). *Cognitive Therapy of Personality Disorders* (2nd ed). New York, NY: Guilford Press.

Beck, A.T., Rush, A.J., Shaw, B.F., & Emery, G. (1979). *Cognitive Therapy of Depression.* New York, NY: Guilford Press.

Beck, J.S. (1995). *Cognitive Therapy Basics and Beyond.* New York, NY: Guilford Press.

Bohart, A.C. (2005). Evidence-based psychotherapy means evidence-informed, not evidence-driven. *Journal of Contemporary Psychotherapy, 35*(1), 39–53.

Bordin, E.S. (1979). The generalizability of the psychoanalytic concept of the working alliance. *Psychotherapy: Theory, Research & Practice, 16*(3), 252.

Clark, D.M. (1986). A cognitive approach to panic. *Behaviour Research and Therapy, 24,* 461–470.

Clark, D.M., & Wells, A. (1995). A cognitive model of social phobia. In R.G. Heimberg, M.R. Liebowitz, D.A. Hope & F.R. Schneier (Eds.). *Social Phobia: Diagnosis, Assessment and Treatment.* New York, NY: Guilford Press.

Colman, A. M. (2015). *A Dictionary of Psychology.* Oxford Quick Reference.

Deacon, B.J., & Farrell, N.R. (2013). Therapist barriers in the dissemination of exposure therapy. In E. Storch, & D. McKay (Eds.), *Treating Variants and Complications in Anxiety Disorders* (pp. 363–373). New York, NY: Springer.

Dudley, R., Kuyken, W., & Padesky, C.A. (2011). Disorder specific and trans-diagnostic case conceptualisation. *Clinical Psychology Review, 31*(2), 213–224.

Duncan, B. L., Miller, S. D., Wampold, B. E., & Hubble, M. A. (Eds.). (2010). *The Heart and Soul of Change: Delivering What Works in Therapy (2nd ed.).* Washington, DC, US: American Psychological Association.

Egan, S. J., Wade, T. D., & Shafran, R. (2011). Perfectionism as a transdiagnostic process: A clinical review. *Clinical Psychology Review, 31*(2), 203–212.

Fairburn, C. G. (2008). *Cognitive Behavior Therapy and Eating Disorders.* Guilford Press.

Fairburn, C. G., Cooper, Z., & Shafran, R. (2003). Cognitive behaviour therapy for eating disorders: A "transdiagnostic" theory and treatment. *Behaviour Research and Therapy, 41*(5), 509–528.

Farchione, T.J., Fairholme, C.P., Ellard, K.K., Boisseau, C.L., Thompson-Hollands, J., Carl, J.R., Gallagher, M.W., Barlow, D.H. (2012). Unified protocol for transdiagnostic treatment of emotional disorders: A randomized controlled trial. *Behavior Therapy, 43*(3), 666–678.

Freeman, A. (1992). Developing treatment conceptualizations in cognitive therapy. In A. Freeman & F. Dattilio (Eds.), *Casebook of Cognitive-Behavior Therapy* (pp. 13–23). New York, NY: Plenum Press.

Freeman, A., & McCloskey, R.D. (2006). Impediments to effective psychotherapy. In R.L. Leahy (Eds.), *Roadblocks in Cognitive-Behavioral Therapy* (pp. 24–48). New York, NY: Guilford Press.

Glasziou, P. (2005). Evidence based medicine: Does it make a difference? Make it evidence informed practice with a little wisdom. *British Medical Journal, 330*(7482), 92.

Grant, A., Mills, J., Mulhern, R., & Short, N. (2004). The therapeutic alliance and case formulation. In A. Grant, J. Mills, R. Mulhern, & N. Short (Eds.), *Cognitive Behavioral Therapy in Mental Health Care* (pp. 7–20). London, England: SAGE.

Greenberger, D., & Padesky, C.A. (1995). *Mind Over Mood: Change How You Feel by Changing the Way you Think.* New York, NY: Guilford Press.

Grove, W. M., Zald, D. H., Lebow, B. S., Snitz, B. E., & Nelson, C. (2000). Clinical versus mechanical prediction: a meta-analysis. *Psychological Assessment, 12*(1), 19.

Hallam, R.S. (2013). *Individual Case Formulation.* Oxford, England: Elsevier.

Harris, R. (2007). *The Happiness Trap: Stop Struggling, Start Living.* Australia: Exisle Publishing.

Harvey, A.G., Watkins, E., Mansell, W, & Shafran, R. (2004). *Cognitive Behavioural Processes Across Psychological Disorders: A Transdiagnostic Approach to Research and Treatment.* New York, NY: Oxford University Press.

Hayes, S.C., Strosahl, K.D., & Wilson, K.G. (2011). *Acceptance and Commitment Therapy: The Process and Practice of Mindful Change.* Guilford Press.

Hayes, S. C., Wilson, K. G., Gifford, E. V., Follette, V. M., & Strosahl, K. (1996). Experiential avoidance and behavioral disorders: A functional dimensional approach to diagnosis and treatment. *Journal of Consulting and Clinical Psychology, 64(6),* 1152–1168.

Horvath, A.O., & Greenberg, L.S. (1989). Development and validation of the Working Alliance Inventory. *Journal of Counseling Psychology, 36*(2), 223.

Horvath, A.O., & Symonds, B.D. (1991). Relation between working alliance and outcome in psychotherapy: A meta-analysis. *Journal of Counseling Psychology, 38*(2), 139–149.

Ingram, R. E. (1990). Self-focused attention in clinical disorders: Review and a conceptual model. *Psychological Bulletin, 107,*156–176.

Johns, R.G., Barkham, M., Kellett, S., & Saxon, D. (2018). A systematic review of therapist effects: A critical narrative update and refinement to review. *Clinical Psychology Review, 67,* 78–93.

Kazantzis, N., Dattilio, F.M., & Dobson, K.S. (2017). *The therapeutic relationship in Cognitive-Behavioral Therapy.* New York, NY: Guilford Press.

Kazantzis, N., Deane, F.P., & Ronan, K.R. (2000). Homework assignments in cognitive and behavioral therapy: A meta-analysis. *Clinical Psychology: Science and Practice, 7*(2), 189–202.

Kim, D. M., Wampold, B. E., & Bolt, D. M. (2006). Therapist effects in psychotherapy: A random-effects modeling of the National Institute of Mental Health Treatment of Depression Collaborative Research Program data. *Psychotherapy Research, 16*(02), 161–172.

Leahy, R.L. (2006). Emotional schemas and resistance. In R.L. Leahy (Ed.), *Roadblocks in Cognitive-Behavioral Therapy* (pp. 91–115). New York, NY: Guilford Press.

Leahy, R.L. (2008). The therapeutic relationship in cognitive–behavioral therapy. *Behavioural and Cognitive Psychotherapy, 36*(6), 769–777.

Lilienfeld, S.O., Ritschel, L.A., Lynn, S.J., Cautin, R.L., & Latzman, R.D. (2013). Why many clinical psychologists are resistant to evidence-based practice: Root causes and constructive remedies. *Clinical Psychology Review, 33*(7), 883–900.

Liotti, G. (1991). Patterns of attachments and the assessment of interpersonal schemata: Understanding and changing difficult patient–therapist relationships in cognitive psychotherapy. *Journal of Cognitive Psychotherapy: An International Quarterly, 5,* 105–113.

Martin, D.J., Garske, J.P., & Davis, K.M. (2000). Relation of the therapeutic alliance with outcome and other variables: a meta-analytic review. *Journal of Consulting and Clinical Psychology, 68,* 438–450.

McEvoy, P.M., & Mahoney, A.E.J. (2013). Intolerance of uncertainty and negative metacognitive beliefs as transdiagnostic mediators of repetitive negative thinking in a clinical sample with anxiety disorders. *Journal of Anxiety Disorders, 27,* 216–224.

McKay, K. M., Imel, Z. E., & Wampold, B. E. (2006). Psychiatrist effects in the psychopharmacological treatment of depression. *Journal of Affective Disorders*, *92*(2–3), 287–290.

Miller, S., Hubble, M., & Duncan, B. (2007). Supershrinks: Why do some therapists clearly stand out above the rest, consistently getting far better results than most of their colleagues? *Psychotherapy Networker*, *31*(6), 26.

Miller, S.D., Duncan, B.L., Brown, J., Sparks, J.A., & Claud, D.A. (2003). The outcome rating scale: A preliminary study of the reliability, validity, and feasibility of a brief visual analog measure. *Journal of Brief Therapy*, *2*(2), 91–100.

Miller, W.R., & Rollnick, S. (2009). Ten things that motivational interviewing is not. *Behavioural and Cognitive Psychotherapy*, *37*(2), 129–140.

Miller, W.R., & Rollnick, S. (2012). *Motivational Interviewing: Helping People Change*. New York, NY: Guilford press.

Moyers, T.B., & Rollnick, S. (2002). A motivational interviewing perspective on resistance in psychotherapy. *Journal of Clinical Psychology*, *58*(2), 185–193.

Needleman, L.D. (2006). Case conceptualization in preventing and responding to therapeutic difficulties. In R.L. Leahy (Eds.), *Roadblocks in Cognitive-Behavioral Therapy* (pp. 3–23). New York, NY: Guilford Press.

Persons, J.B. (1989). *Cognitive Therapy in Practice: A Case Formulation Approach*. New York, NY: Norton.

Persons, J.B., & Tompkins, M.A. (2007). Cognitive-behavioral case formulation. In T.D. Eells (Ed.), *Handbook of Psychotherapy Case Formulation* (2nd ed.). New York, NY: Guilford Press.

Prochaska, J.O., & DiClemente, C. (1983). Stages and processes of self-change of smoking: toward an integrative model of change. *Journal of Consulting and Clinical Psychology*, *51*, 390–395.

Rouf, K., Fennel, M., Westbrook, D., Cooper, M., & Bennett-Levy, J. (2004). Devising effective behavioural experiments. In J. Bennett-Levy, G. Butler, M. Fennell, A. Hackmann, M. Mueller, & D. Westbrook (Eds.). *Oxford Guide to Behavioural Experiments in Cognitive Therapy*. Oxford, England: Oxford University Press.

Safran, J.D. (1998). *Widening the Scope of Cognitive Therapy: the Therapeutic Relationship, Emotion and the Process of Change.* Northvale, NJ: Aronson.

Safran, J.D., & Muran, J.C. (2000). *Negotiating the Therapeutic Alliance: A Relational Treatment Guide.* New York, NY: Guilford Press.

Safran, J.D., & Segal, L.S. (1990). *Interpersonal Process in Cognitive Therapy.* New York, NY: Basic Books.

Safran, J.D., Muran, J.C., Samstag, L.W., & Stevens, C. (2002). Repairing alliance ruptures. In J. R. Norcross (Ed.), *Psychotherapy Relationships That Work* (pp. 235–254). New York, NY: Oxford University Press.

Salkovskis, P.M. (1989). Somatic problems. In K. Hawton, P.M. Salkovskis, J. Kirk, & D.M. Clark (Eds.) *Cognitive Behaviour Therapy for Psychiatric Problems: A Practical Guide* (pp. 235–276). Oxford, England: Oxford University Press.

Salkovskis, P.M., Forrester, E., & Richards, C. (1998). Cognitive–behavioural approach to understanding obsessional thinking. *British Journal of Psychiatry, 173(Suppl 35),* 53–63.

Schmidt, U., Startup, H., & Treasure, J. (2018). *A Cognitive-Interpersonal Therapy Workbook for Treating Anorexia Nervosa: The Maudsley Model.* London, England: Taylor and Francis.

Shapiro, D. A., & Shapiro, D. (1982). Meta-analysis of comparative therapy outcome studies: a replication and refinement. *Psychological Bulletin, 92*(3), 581.

Tompkins, M.A. (1999). Using a case formulation to manage treatment nonresponse. *Journal of Cognitive Psychotherapy, 13,* 317–330.

Tompkins, M.A. (2006). Effective homework. In R.L. Leahy (Ed.), *Roadblocks in Cognitive-Behavioral Therapy* (pp. 49–66). New York, NY: Guilford Press.

Treasure, J., & Schmidt, U. (2013). The cognitive-interpersonal maintenance model of anorexia nervosa revisited: a summary of the evidence for cognitive, socio-emotional and interpersonal predisposing and perpetuating factors. *Journal of Eating Disorders, 1,* 13–22.

Vansteenkiste, M., Williams, G.C., & Resnicow, K. (2012). Toward systematic integration between self-determination theory and motivational interviewing as examples of top-down and bottom-up intervention development: Autonomy or volition as a fundamental theoretical principle. *International Journal of Behavioral Nutrition and Physical Activity, 9*(1), 23.

Vlaeyen, J.W.S., & Linton, S.J. (2002). Pain-related fear and its consequences in chronic musculoskeletal pain. In S.J. Linton (Ed.), *New Avenues for the Prevention of Chronic Musculoskeletal Pain and Disability* (pp. 81–103). Amsterdam, The Netherlands: Elsevier Science.

Waller, G. (2009). Evidence-based treatment and therapist drift. *Behaviour Research and Therapy, 47*, 119–127.

Waller, G. (2012). The myths of motivation: time for a fresh look at some received wisdom in the eating disorders? *International Journal of Eating Disorders, 45*(1), 1–16.

Waller, G. (2016). Treatment protocols for eating disorders: Clinicians' attitudes, concerns, adherence and difficulties delivering evidence-based psychological interventions. *Current Psychiatry Reports, 18*, 36. doi: 10.1007/s11920-016-0679-0

Waller, G., & Turner, H. (2016). Therapist drift redux: why well-meaning clinicians fail to deliver evidence-based therapy, and how to get back on track. *Behaviour Research and Therapy, 77*, 129–37.

Wampold, B.E. (2001). *The Great Psychotherapy Debate: Model, Methods, and Findings.* Mahwah, NJ: Lawrence Erlbaum.

Wampold, B.E. (2006). The psychotherapist. In J.C. Norcross, L.E. Beutler & R.F. Levant (Eds.), *Evidence-based Practices in Mental Health: Debate and Dialogues on the Fundamental Questions* (pp. 200–208). Washington, DC: American Psychological Association.

Wampold, B. E. (2007). Psychotherapy: The humanistic (and effective) treatment. *American Psychologist, 62*, 857– 873. doi:10.1037/0003-066X.62.8.857

Warwick, H.M., & Salkovskis, P.M. (1990). Hypochondriasis. *Behaviour Research and Therapy, 28*, 105–117.

Wells, A. (2005). Detached mindfulness in cognitive therapy: a metacognitive analysis and ten techniques. *Journal of Rational-Emotive & Cognitive-Behavior Therapy, 23*, 337–355.

Wells, A. (2006). Anxiety disorders, metacognition, and change. In R.L. Leahy (Eds.), *Roadblocks in Cognitive-Behavioral Therapy* (pp. 69–90). New York, NY: Guilford Press.

Wells, A., & Clark, D.M. (1997). Social phobia: A cognitive approach. In G.C.L. Davey (Ed.), *Phobias: A Handbook of Theory, Research and Treatment* (pp. 3–26). Chichester, England: Wiley.

Westra, H.A., & Dozois, D.J. (2006). Preparing clients for cognitive behavioral therapy: A randomized pilot study of motivational interviewing for anxiety. *Cognitive Therapy and Research, 30*(4), 481–498.

Westra, H.A., Aviram, A., & Doell, F.K. (2011). Extending motivational interviewing to the treatment of major mental health problems: current directions and evidence. *The Canadian Journal of Psychiatry, 56*(11), 643–650.

Wilson G.T. (1996). Manual-based treatments: The clinical application of research findings. *Behaviour Research and Therapy, 34*, 295–314.

Woodruff-Borden, J., Brothers, A. J., & Lister, S. C. (2001). Self-focused attention: Commonalities across psychopathologies and predictors. *Behavioural and Cognitive Psychotherapy, 29*(2), 169–178.

Wright, J.H., & Davis, D. (1994). The therapeutic relationship in cognitive-behavioral therapy: Patient perceptions and therapist responses. *Cognitive and Behavioral Practice, 1*(1), 25–45.

Young, J.E., Klosko, J.S., & Weishaar, M. (2003). *Schema Therapy: A Practitioner's Guide*. New York, NY: Guilford Press.

# APPENDIX A

**Four Visual Analogue Scales for Assessing Willingness**

Target Goal or Exercise:

.............................................................................................................

1. **Benefits** (what good am I likely to get?)

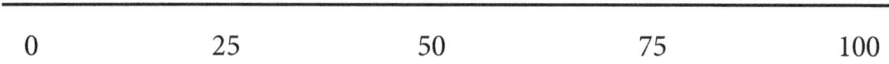

---

| 0 | 25 | 50 | 75 | 100 |

2. **Costs** (but what will it cost me?)

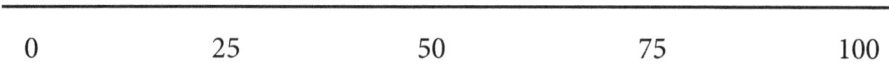

---

| 0 | 25 | 50 | 75 | 100 |

3. Alignment with my **Values** (to what degree will this action bring me closer to the Life I wish for myself; or help me be the person I want to be?)

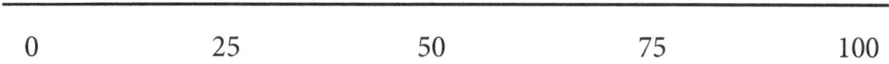

---

| 0 | 25 | 50 | 75 | 100 |

4. Confidence that I can do it

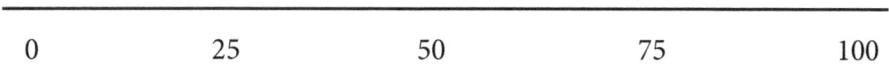

---

| 0 | 25 | 50 | 75 | 100 |

So, given my ratings on COSTS and CONFIDENCE, what might I need to work on, so that I am more willing to make this change?

.............................................................................................................
.............................................................................................................
.............................................................................................................
.............................................................................................................

# APPENDIX B

## Layers of Cognition — Blank Client Worksheet

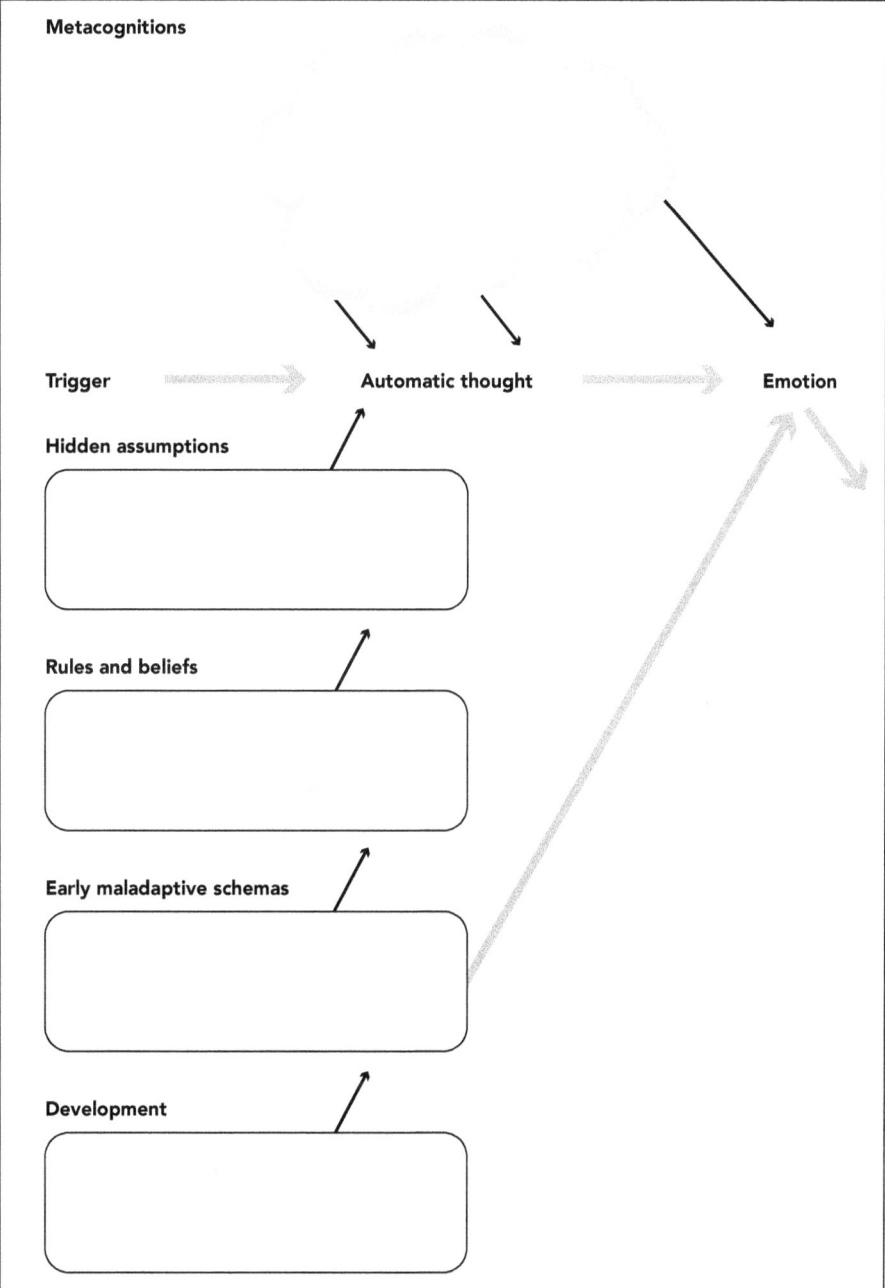

**Metacognitions**

**Trigger** ⟹ **Automatic thought** ⟹ **Emotion**

**Hidden assumptions**

**Rules and beliefs**

**Early maladaptive schemas**

**Development**

# APPENDIX C

## Worksheet to Practice Identifying Cognitions

*Retraining Exercise for Noticing Hidden Assumptions*

Many people find that their mind automatically interprets events and sees situations in all-or-nothing and black-and-white ways. The potential problem with this type of thinking is that it can lead to feelings of inadequacy, unnecessary stress and even hopelessness.

This exercise starts with some examples from others for you to see and work with. The second part is for you to notice a few each day and do the same re-writing. It takes practice. If done frequently enough, the practice will really retrain the automatic processes of your mind.

| The automatic thought | The hidden all-or-nothing implication | A more realistic and helpful option |
| --- | --- | --- |
| If I praise myself, that would mean I am arrogant and one of those people that others hate. | You are either humble and nice, or conceited and bad; all acknowledgement of hard work is terrible. | It's okay for anyone to privately acknowledge when they've done okay. I would not think this same thought about a friend. |
| I am so ashamed of that report after getting some negative feedback. | My work should be flawless; any criticism means I have not done well enough. Getting help means you are not good enough. | Some criticism is inevitable in life and it can help a person grow and develop. It is not possible or necessary to go through life without making any mistakes or getting help. |
| Those people must be thinking I'm such an idiot because I'm SO nervous and I can't even relax at a birthday party. | I'm good at reading others' minds; anxiety is highly visible; when people perceive anxiety, they think nasty judgmental thoughts; all people think the same. | I don't know what they are thinking; they probably are not thinking about me at all. The more I focus on how anxious I feel and look, the worse I feel. I'll try a conversation. |

# APPENDIX D

## Part A. Client Handout on How to Learn Cognitive Therapy

*Where do my bad feelings come from?*
*The Cognitive Theory of distress and dysfunction*

Most of our emotions arise from different types of thoughts or cognitions. Our thoughts about an event or situation have a much greater influence on our emotions than the situation itself. This is why four people exposed to the same situation or event may all have different reactions.

Some cognitions are fleeting and automatic (in the moment), while others are stable and remain the same over many years. This table illustrates the most common examples of cognitions.

| Automatic Thoughts | Hidden Thoughts | Underlying Stable Beliefs |
| --- | --- | --- |
| interpretations | Assumptions | Conditional Beliefs (I'll be accepted if...) |
| conclusions | Implications | Core Beliefs (I'm defective; or people hurt you) |
| comparisons | Rules | Rules (mistakes are unforgiveable) |
| visual images | Old and familiar beliefs | Beliefs about our thoughts (worry helps me) |
| worry about future | | |
| ruminating on past | | |

Our thoughts have the following qualities; they:

- are automatic; we do not try to have most thoughts, but our mind produces them.

- are not necessarily accurate; or at least only partly accurate.

- are not always helpful; even if accurate, they make us feel bad for no gain.

- feel true at the time.

If we mistake a thought that we have as a fact, we will be pushed around by painful emotions and we may engage in actions that are unproductive. By learning to notice the automatic thinking content that our mind produces, we can learn to step back from unhelpful or inaccurate thoughts and to have more stable emotions.

*How can we get better at noticing our thoughts if they are automatic, hidden and feel true?*

1. **Monitoring.** Make a written or electronic record of the main emotions that cause you distress. Every time you catch that emotion in your mind, pause and start to observe things about that emotional state. Without judging it, be curious about where that emotion sits in your body, what urges might accompany that emotion and (crucially) what thoughts were running through your mind just prior to or during that emotion. Writing out these observations is much more effective than mental note-taking.

2. **Deliberate observation.** Stop and try to do nothing, then notice any thoughts that your mind automatically generates for you. A great example might be to sit with eyes shut and count 20 breaths, trying to keep 100% of your attention on the small detail of every single breath. It is inevitable that your mind will involuntarily produce cognitions, even while you are trying not to think. Your job is to notice these thoughts as the curious observer without judging the thoughts as good or bad; nor trying to make them go away; nor attending to them.

Let's look at some real-people examples. In each case, are these sentences facts or 'cognitions'?

If cognitions, then what sort (assumptions, imagery, predictions, comparisons, rules, thoughts)?

When **Maria** realises that she has sent the wrong attachment in an email to work colleagues, she feels really disappointed with herself then super-anxious about what those colleagues will think of her. She imagines people chuckling at her mistake and finds herself thinking, 'I am such an idiot. What a stupid mistake. I will never live this down'.

**Andrew** is taking his time in the storeroom at work because his team are all about to head out to lunch for their end-of-month lunch out of the office. He has his usual thoughts: 'I hate these socials. I have nothing to say and it gets so awkward. I can't afford for these people to see how useless and anxious I am. It will be so humiliating'.

| Emotion or Feeling | Immediate cognitive content and process | Indirect factors: beliefs and past experiences |
| --- | --- | --- |
| Fear or anxiety | Perception of threat; assuming there is some danger; predicting a bad outcome | Past experiences. Assumptions about likelihood of the occurrence and how disastrous it would be ('cost') |
| Worry | Predictions about what threats may arise in the future<br><br>Beliefs about the helpfulness of worry | Assumptions about likelihood, potential disastrousness or cost, underestimations about one's ability to cope. Intolerance of uncertainty |
| Worthlessness; uselessness | Self-criticism; judging oneself negatively against a high standard | Core beliefs such as 'I'm not good enough' |
| Pessimism; despair; hopelessness | Thoughts and assumptions that nothing can change | Past experiences<br>Lack of knowledge of or access to resources to get help<br>Lack of problem-solving skills |
| Guilt | Judging oneself for doing something that is wrong (with the assumption that we were responsible and able to create a better outcome) | Core beliefs about self<br>Strict rules about right and wrong |
| Shame | Assuming that others see us as a bad person or having done something terrible | Past experiences of trauma<br>Our core beliefs about morality and the importance of what others think<br>One of our parents used guilt or shaming as a parenting style |
| Self-directed anger | Violation of expectations, where high standards have been set for oneself. All-or-nothing thinking | Core beliefs (e.g. about right-wrong and personal entitlement)<br>A critical parenting style that we have internalised |
| Resentment | A particular form of thinking that things could be and should be different or fairer | History of injustices. Core beliefs (e.g. about right-wrong and personal entitlement) |

## Part B. A Brief Formula for Thought Challenging

A. Notice and label the emotion(s). Notice as the curious, non-judging observer.

B. Look for the thoughts, assumptions, predictions, interpretations, comparisons etc... (cognitions) giving rise to each feeling. Work with the assumption that many of my thoughts are inaccurate and unhelpful — even the ones that FEEL true.

C. Try to challenge these thoughts using these (learned) questions:

1. Is my mind over-estimating the likelihood of the dreaded things actually happening? Do I actually know or have evidence — or is my mind wanting to assume the worst?

   What would I say to someone else if they told me they were thinking this way?

2. Is my mind over-estimating how disastrous (the cost) it would be if that feared thing did happen? Do I actually know or have evidence?

   What would I say to someone else if they told me they were thinking this way?

3. Is my mind under-estimating how well I could cope if that dreaded thing actually happened? Do I actually know or have evidence?

   What would I say to someone else if they told me they were thinking this way?

4. Is my mind trying to allocate too much time to this? When should I work on it? And how and for how long should I allocate that time?

5. What evidence does my mind use to support the negative or worrying feeling? And is that evidence reliable and relevant to this situation?

6. What evidence is there already that it may not work out that way?

7. Could I test this out somehow to gather more disproving evidence? What safe test could I do?

8. Am I making one of my usual thinking errors (all-or-nothing; unrealistic standards; intolerance of uncertainty; wanting more certainty than is possible or necessary; selective filtering, catastrophizing, mind-reading, personalising …)?

9. What are my healthy guidelines or principles that I try to follow in these situations?

D. Arrive at a new way of thinking. Write it out. Can I enact this more helpful thought or test it out somehow?

E. Check in. So now…

- How should I be thinking from now on?
- How could I be feeling right now?
- What is the wisest course of action to take?
- What will happen if I do not take that wiser action now?
- What will I say to myself the next 30 times my mind tries to distress me about this?
- How much time ought I allocate to this issue from now on? And IF I was to work on it anymore, then when and how?

## Part C. Practicing Cognitive Therapy at an Effective Level

Here are some principles to keep in mind:

- Anyone can learn and use cognitive therapy – it is universal – as long as you are willing to put some work in.

- Cognitive therapy is not a natural way to think – it takes practice. Nobody is good at it to start with. But, if you do daily practice, it is almost inevitable that you will get good at it.

- It takes most people somewhere between 2 and 4 months to feel that they have mastered cognitive therapy and that it starts to be an automatic process in their own repertoire. In the meanwhile, it feels effortful and a bit contrived or unnatural.

- There is a dose-dependent effect. That is, the more effort you apply and the harder you hit the emotion, the better effect you will get. It is much like trying to treat a headache. If you take one Panadol you will get a certain result and it might or might not be enough. If you take two Panadol plus water plus a stretch and then another two tablets two six hours later, you will get a different result.

- You can increase the 'dose' of cognitive therapy by allocating a certain amount of time to it, reading some guidelines so you get the technique right, writing it out (it is weaker if you do it in your head), and consider sharing it with someone.

- Think about what outcome you want to have in 6 months from now and be confident that the effort you put in every day is in line with that outcome. How will it feels in 6 months from now if you know you have given yourself a half dose? How will it feel if you know you've applied yourself as well as you can?

- Do daily exercises. If you wanted to learn any new skill or technique, it makes sense to do drills over and over in a structured learning environment instead of waiting until a crisis when you need to suddenly apply those skills.

- Skill acquisition always follows certain pathways such as:
  - Orientation and familiarisation

- Skill acquisition
- Skill practice
- Skill mastery
- Skill application

Cognitive therapy is no different, so generate some daily exercises with your therapist.

# APPENDIX E

## Example of a Behavioural Experiment Worksheet

THE FEAR OR PREDICTION THAT I AM TESTING: ....................................................................

....................................................................................................................................................

....................................................................................................................................................

....................................................................................................................................................

MY DELIBERATE EXPERIMENTAL ACTION: ..........................................................................

....................................................................................................................................................

....................................................................................................................................................

....................................................................................................................................................

....................................................................................................................................................

....................................................................................................................................................

| SCARY PREDICTIONS THAT MY MIND MAKES: THOUGHTS, IMAGERY, ASSUMPTIONS (RATE LIKELIHOOD %) | ACTUAL OBSERVED OUTCOME |
|---|---|
| .............................................................. | .............................................................. |
| .............................................................. | .............................................................. |
| .............................................................. | .............................................................. |
| .............................................................. | .............................................................. |
| .............................................................. | .............................................................. |

CONCLUSIONS AND LESSONS (What I can now think, and do and feel): .....................................

....................................................................................................................................................

....................................................................................................................................................

....................................................................................................................................................

FUTURE TESTS: .........................................................................................................................

....................................................................................................................................................

....................................................................................................................................................

# Appendix F

## Client Worksheet for the End of Each Consultation

*End-of-Session Summary*                    *Date:.........................*

1. What we worked on today that I want to remember.

2. What tasks did we agree for me to do before the next appointment?

3. What specific and achievable goals I want to set for myself until the next appointment?

4. What will I be monitoring this week (e.g. behaviours, urges, thoughts, feelings etc.)?

5. What topic(s) do I want to get onto next appointment?

*SRS items:*

6. To what degree (0 to 5) did we work on and talk about what I wanted to work on and talk about? .........

   Comments: ................................................................................................

   ................................................................................................

7. To what degree (0 to 5) did I feel heard, understood and respected? .........

   Comments: ................................................................................................

   ................................................................................................

8. To what degree (0 to 5) was today's session right for me? .........

   Comments: ................................................................................................

   ................................................................................................

# Appendix G

## Handout for Clients on Effective Therapy

### THE SEVEN PILLARS OF EFFECTIVE THERAPY

1. **Goals**. Have defined and achievable and measurable goals that you would like to aim for. Pick one or two at a time: too many goals dilute the dose of therapy that you get. Your therapist will ask you what your goals are at the start of therapy.

2. **Consistency**. Keep working on the same one or two goals. Chopping and changing does not help.

3. **Shared Strategy**. We need to develop a clear systematic or strategic approach to work towards those goals of yours. The psychologist and client need to agree on what is the nature of the problem and what is maintaining that problem. Equally, you will need a shared understanding about why a certain treatment will work. Ask your therapist how the treatment will work for you and discuss any differences of opinion.

4. **Internalise Responsibility**. Your therapist can help with guidance, adding levels of understanding and offering direction. They will work hard to arrive at the best treatment approach for you. It is the client's responsibility to (a) contribute to the assessment process, (b) contribute to the setting of clear, achievable goals, (c) contribute to an agenda for each session and stick to that agenda, (d) attempt the prescribed tasks between each consultation, and (e) take the other steps that are required to reach your goals.

5. **Willingness To Have Some Negative Emotions**. Change nearly always leads to discomfort. So, if change is what we want to achieve, then we must find some willingness to tolerate discomfort and test out our fears. One of the most helpful sources of willingness is to reflect on how important this change is to you. If something is aligned with your values for how you want to live your life or see yourself as a person, then you tend to be determined to achieve that and so your willingness to do scary or hard work increases. With your therapist, discuss your

motivational levels and how to increase them. Discuss how to make any discomfort more tolerable – you may wish to learn some distress-tolerance and mood-regulation skills early in the therapy.

6. **Confidence.** It is important that you have a reasonable degree of confidence that you can work on your goals. If your confidence is low – don't let that stop you. The best thing to do is talk about that with your therapist and work out ways to increase your confidence (like setting smaller steps or goals and increasing your coping skills first).

7. **Trust.** It is very important that you feel that your therapist is interested in you and your outcome and that you trust them to manage your interests and issues with care and confidentiality. If there is a breach in that relationship, do try to talk about it with the psychologist, as it can usually be addressed successfully.

**so, signs of ineffective therapy would include...**

Having no clear goals that remain consistent over time, having no agreed method to achieve those goals, having no time-frame to work towards, expecting that the psychologist will fix you (without doing much yourself), and avoiding difficult emotions.

www.ingramcontent.com/pod-product-compliance
Lightning Source LLC
Chambersburg PA
CBHW050717280326
41926CB00088B/3076